PEACEFUL POSES, PEACEFUL MIND

Yoga Techniques to Alleviate Stress for Beginners

CONTENTS

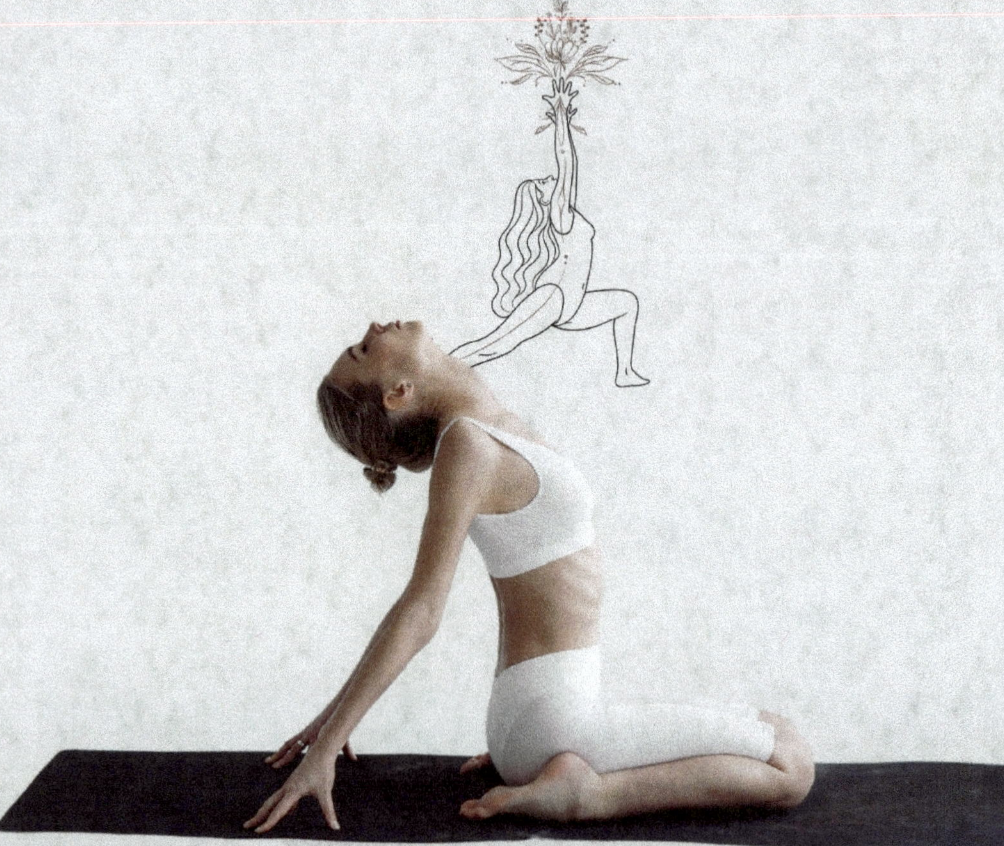

Introduction

Here is a one-paragraph summary for the "Peaceful Poses, Peaceful Mind: Yoga Techniques to Alleviate Stress for Beginners" resource:

In a world filled with constant demands and mounting pressure, the ancient practice of yoga offers a sanctuary of tranquility. "Peaceful Poses, Peaceful Mind" is a beginner's guide to harnessing the stress-relieving benefits of yoga.

Through an exploration of yoga's history and principles, an understanding of how it reduces anxiety, and a curated collection of soothing postures and sequences, this resource equips readers with the knowledge and tools to cultivate greater inner calm. With step-by-step instructions and visual demonstrations, beginners will learn to properly execute each pose while also gaining insight into the physiological and psychological effects.

By shifting inward and developing heightened body awareness, readers will unlock yoga's power to quiet the chattering mind, release muscular tension, and instill a profound sense of serenity - empowering them to navigate life's challenges with greater resilience and composure.

About
Yoga

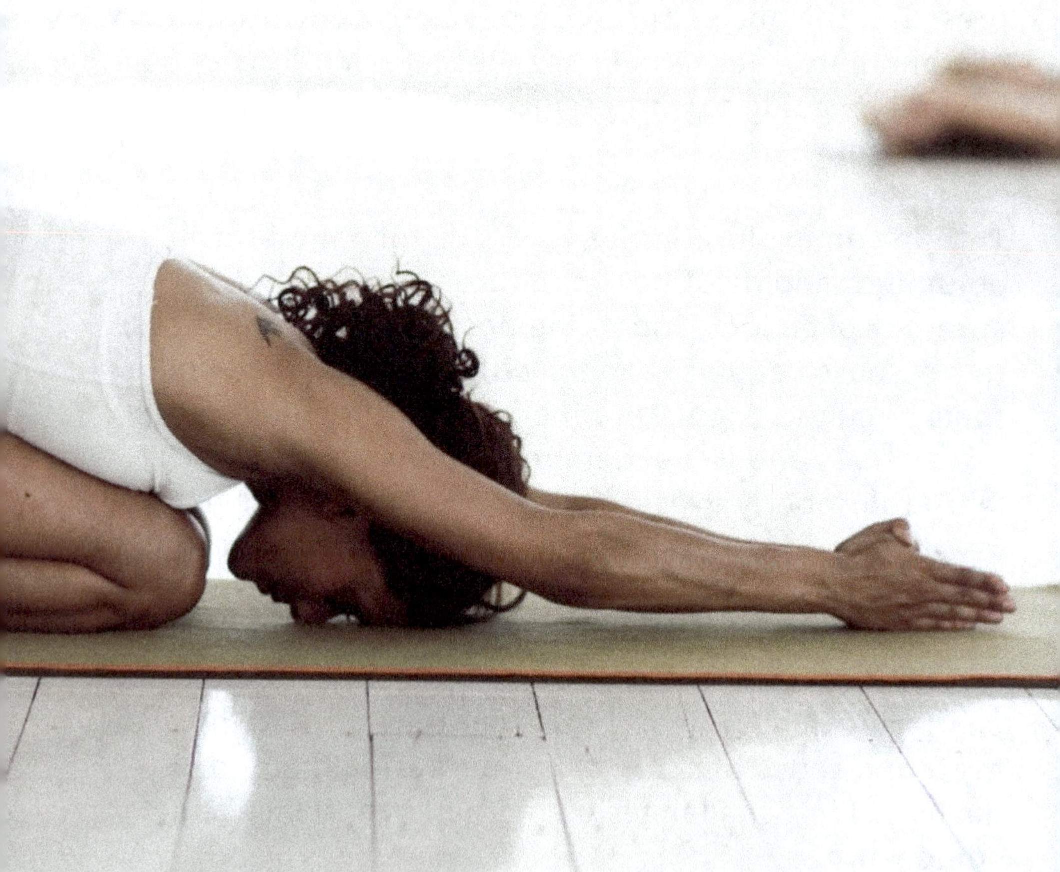

WHAT IS YOGA?

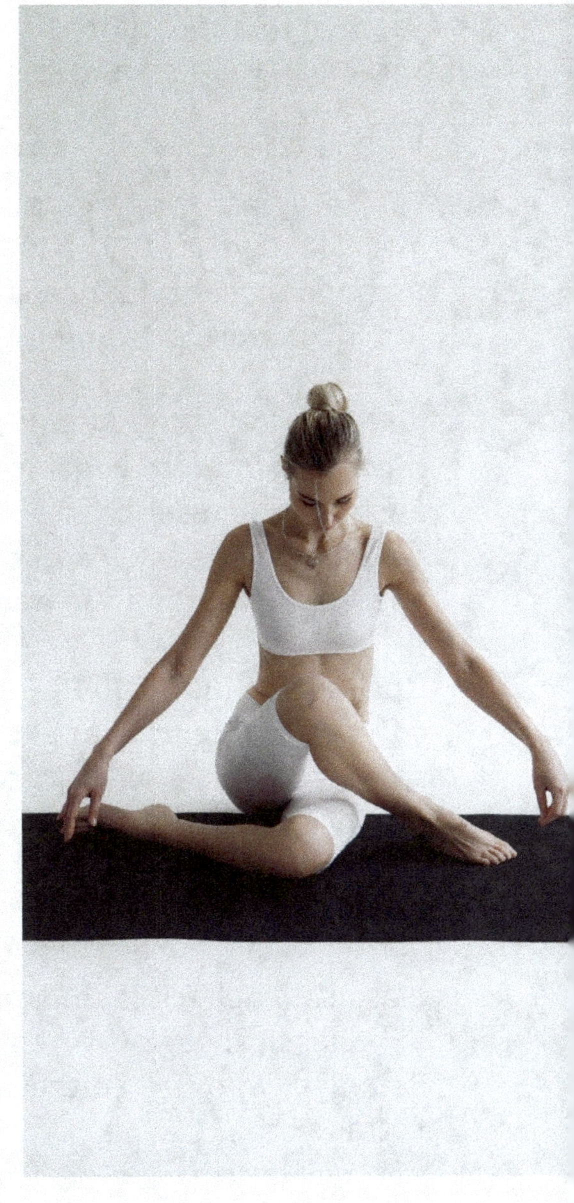

Yoga originated in India thousands of years ago.

Yoga has been closely associated with both physical and spiritual practice, and its traditions have developed over the course of millennia.

This meditative practice tends to combine physical exercise, controlled breathing, and mental exercise that emphasizes mindfulness and unity between body and spirit.

Traditionally, the ultimate goal of yoga has been captured in the term moksha, which might be translated as freedom from samsara, the cycle of death and rebirth.

HISTORICAL ASPECT OF YOGA

The history of yoga is a rich tapestry that spans thousands of years, with its origins deeply rooted in ancient India. Understanding its historical development is essential to appreciate the depth and significance of this practice. Here's an overview of the historical aspects of yoga:

- Early Origins: The origins of yoga can be traced back over 5,000 years to the Indus Valley Civilization. Archaeological evidence suggests that yoga-like practices were prevalent during this time.

- Vedic Period (1500-500 BCE): The earliest written records related to yoga are found in the Vedas, ancient Indian scriptures. Yoga was initially developed as a means of connecting with the divine and understanding the nature of reality.

- Upanishads (800-200 BCE): The Upanishads, a collection of texts that explore the philosophical and spiritual aspects of life, delve deeper into the practice of yoga. They introduce concepts like meditation and the union of the individual soul (Atman) with the universal soul (Brahman).

- Classical Yoga (circa 2nd century BCE – 4th century CE): Classical yoga is often associated with the sage Patanjali, who is credited with compiling the "Yoga Sutras."

This foundational text outlines the eight limbs of yoga, including ethical guidelines (yamas and niyamas), physical postures (asanas), breathing techniques (pranayama), and meditation (dhyana).

- Post-Classical Period (5th century CE – 18th century CE): This era saw the development of various schools of yoga, each with its unique approach and emphasis. For example, Hatha yoga, which focuses on physical postures and breath control, gained popularity during this time.

- Modern Yoga (Late 19th century – Present): The late 19th and 20th centuries witnessed the introduction of yoga to the Western world. Figures like Swami Vivekananda and Paramahansa Yogananda played pivotal roles in popularizing yoga in the West. The practice evolved to accommodate contemporary lifestyles, resulting in various yoga styles, including Vinyasa, Bikram, and Ashtanga.

- Yoga Today: Yoga has become a global phenomenon, with millions of practitioners worldwide. It is not only a physical exercise but also a lifestyle and a philosophy for well-being. Yoga's adaptability and inclusivity have contributed to its enduring popularity.

DIFFERENT STYLES OF YOGA

When you're trying to determine which of the different types of yoga is best for you, remember that there is no right or wrong one— just one that might not be right for you at this moment.

"Like any form of exercise, choose something you want to do," says Stephanie Saunders, executive director of fitness at Beachbody and a certified yoga instructor. "Bikram or Iyengar might appeal to you if you are a very detailed person. If you are more of a free spirit, vinyasa or aerial yoga might be fun. Find a class that makes you excited to go."

So which one will get you excited? Our guide to the common types of yoga can help you decide whether you're in more of a restorative yoga or a power yoga kind of mood, or anything in between.

Kundalini Yoga

Yogi Bhajan, teacher, and spiritual leader, brought this style of yoga to the West in the late 1960s. "Kundalini" in Sanskrit translates to "life force energy" (known as prana or chi in the yoga community), which is thought to be tightly coiled at the base of the spine. These yoga sequences are carefully designed to stimulate or unlock this energy and to reduce stress and negative thinking.

"You get to elevate your consciousness and feel great," says Veronica Parker, an E-RYT 200, and a certified kundalini yoga teacher.

This is accomplished by challenging both mind and body with chanting, singing, meditation, and kriyas (specific series of poses paired with breath work and chanting). You might notice everyone is wearing white, as it's believed to deflect negativity and increase your aura. Typically, a kundalini class starts with a mantra (a focus for the class), then includes breathing exercises, warmups to get the body moving, increasingly more challenging poses, and a final relaxation and meditation, says Parker.

Who Might Like It: Anyone in search of a physical, yet also spiritual practice, or those who like singing or chanting.

Vinyasa Yoga

Vinyasa yoga is also called "flow yoga" or "vinyasa flow". It is an incredibly common style. One example is 3 Week Yoga Retreat's flow yoga for beginners. It was adapted from the more regimented ashtanga practice a couple of decades ago.

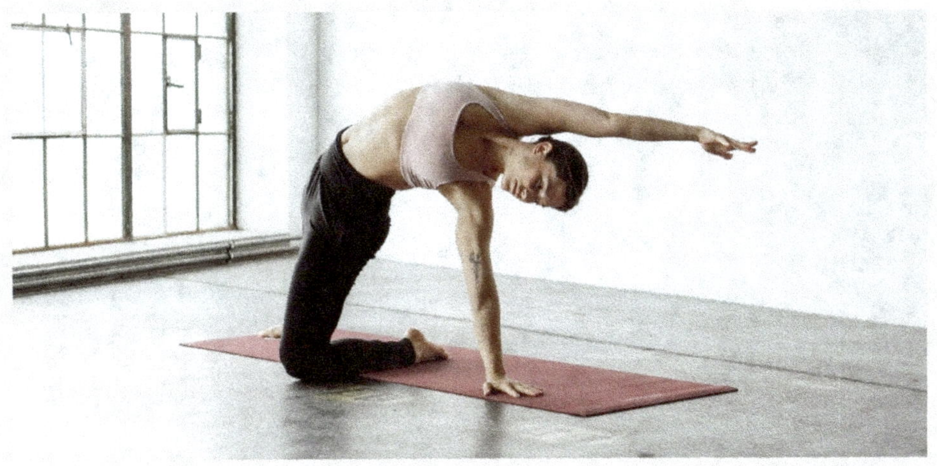

The word "vinyasa" translates to "place in a special way," which is often interpreted as linking breath and movement. You'll often see words like slow, dynamic, or mindful paired with vinyasa or flow to indicate the intensity of a practice.

"Vinyasa flow is a style of yoga where the poses are synchronized with the breath in a continuous rhythmic flow," says Sherrell Moore-Tucker, RYT 200. "The flow can be meditative in nature, calming the mind and nervous system, even though you're moving."

Vinyasa yoga is suitable for those who've never tried yoga as well as those who've been practicing for years.

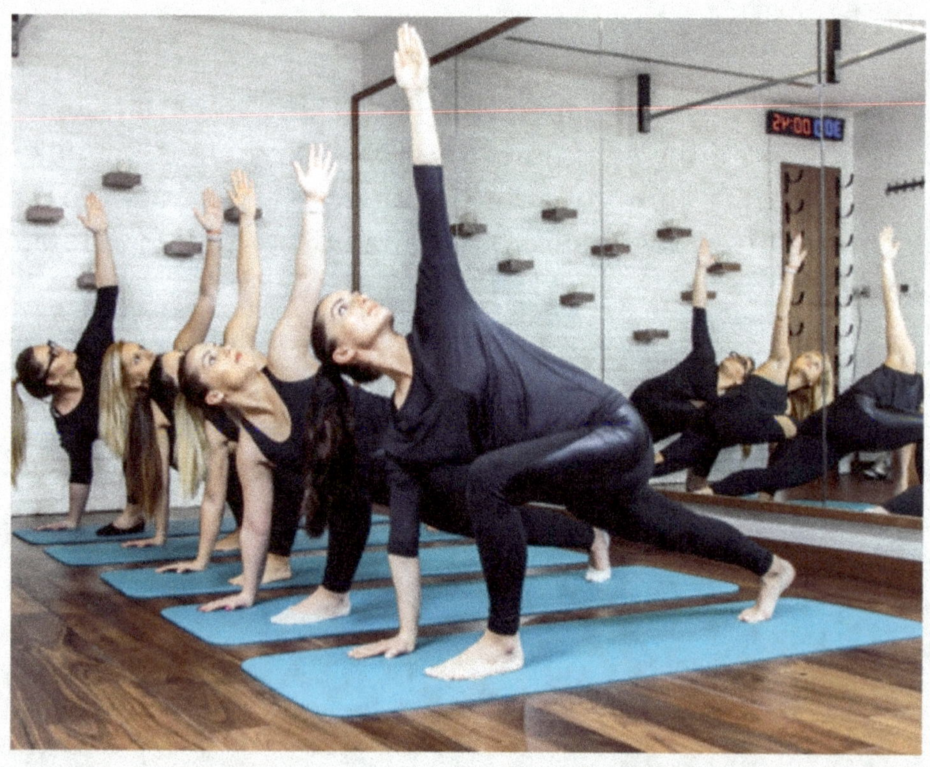

Who Might Like It: Anyone who wants more movement and less stillness from their yoga practice.

Hatha Yoga

Hatha yoga derives its name from the Sanskrit words for sun and moon, and it's designed to balance opposing forces. The balance in hatha yoga might come from strength and flexibility, physical and mental energy, or breath and the body. "Hatha is a blanket term for many different 'styles' and schools that use the body as a means for self-inquiry," says Jennifer Campbell-Overbeeke, E-RYT 500.

It's often used as a catch-all term for the physical side of yoga, is more traditional in nature, or is billed as yoga for beginners. "Hatha translates to 'forceful,' but this relates more to the aspect of concentration and regularity of practice rather than applying unnecessary force to the body," says Campbell-Overbeeke.

To be considered hatha, classes must include a mix of asana (poses), pranayama (breathing exercises), and meditation, so other types of yoga — like Iyengar, ashtanga, or Bikram — are technically considered to be hatha yoga as well.

Who Might Like It: Anyone looking for a balanced practice, or those in search of a gentler type of yoga.

Ashtanga Yoga

Ashtanga yoga consists of six series of specific poses taught in order. Each pose and each series is "given" to a student when their teacher decides they have mastered the previous one. This is a very physical, flow-style yoga with spiritual components — you might remember it as the type Madonna did in the late '90s. Ashtanga teachers give hands-on adjustments, and in Mysore-style studios (named after the city where the practice's guru, Sri K. Pattabhi Jois, lived and taught), each student has a unique practice.

"The practitioner moves at the pace of her own breath and to her personal edge, or growth point," says Lara Land, a level two authorized ashtanga teacher. "Each person memorizes the practice and moves at her own pace through the poses."

Ashtanga vinyasa yoga is often taught as "led" classes in the West, where the first or second series is taught from start to finish over the course of 90 minutes to two hours. There is no music played in ashtanga classes.

Who Might Like It: Anyone who likes routine or a more physical yet spiritual practice.

Yin Yoga

Yin yoga is a slower style of yoga in which poses are held for a minute and eventually up to five minutes or more. It is a type of yoga with roots in martial arts as well as yoga, and it's designed to increase circulation in the joints and improve flexibility.

The practice focuses on the hips, lower back, and thighs and uses props like bolsters, blankets, and blocks to let gravity do the work, helping to relax. While other forms of yoga focus on the major muscle groups, yin yoga targets the body's connective tissues.

Yin also aids recovery from hard workouts. "Adding a deep stretch and holding class like yin can be extremely beneficial to a strong body," says Megan Kearney, a Yoga Medicine instructor. Holding poses longer benefits the mind as well as the body, providing a chance to practice being still. "This is a beautiful practice that honors stillness," says Moore-Tucker. "This style of practice is a great balance for vinyasa flow."

Who Might Like It: Those who need to stretch out after a tough workout, or anyone interested in a slower-paced practice.

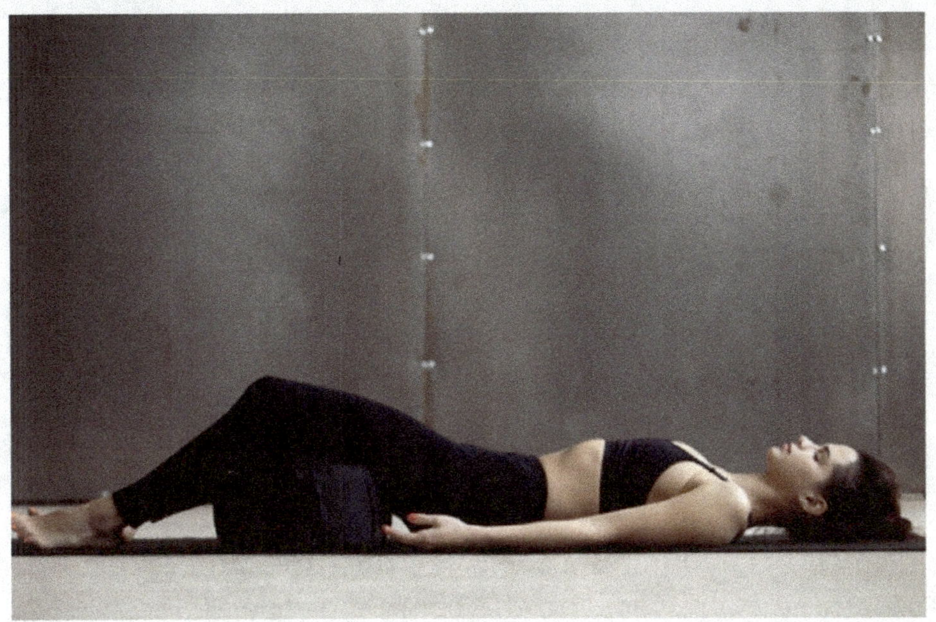

Iyengar Yoga

Named for its founder, B.K.S. Iyengar, who developed his classical, alignment-based practice in India. This type of yoga became popular in the US in the 1970s. Iyengar yoga is known for the high level of training required of its teachers and for its resourceful use of props. While considered optional in many practices, multiple props are used in Iyengar classes — including chairs, walls, and benches, in addition to more common ones like straps, blocks, and bolsters.

Paul Keoni Chun, an E-RYT 200, likes this more static form of yoga for older adults, since it "emphsizes detailed alignment and longer holds of positions." Iyengar yoga is usually less intense than other types of yoga, although that can vary based on the instructor or class. But generally, it's suitable for people of all ages and skill levels.

Who Might Like It: Someone who likes detailed instruction, anyone with physical limitations, or those in search of a more classical form of yoga.

Bikram Yoga

Bikram Choudhury developed Bikram yoga. It is a form of hot yoga. These classes, like ashtanga classes, consist of a set series of poses performed in the same order, and the practice has strict rules.

Each class is 90 minutes, with 26 postures and two breathing exercises, and the room must be 105° Fahrenheit with 40 percent humidity.

Additionally, instructors do not adjust students.

Since Bikram yoga has so many rules, many studios simply call their classes "hot yoga" so they can customize their offerings. Devotees of hot yoga tout the massive amount of sweat and the added flexibility the practice gives them.

"Practicing yoga in a heated environment allows students to get deeper into postures, improves circulation, and aids in detoxifying the body," says Natalie Sleik, RYT 200, who teaches hot power yoga.

Who Might Like It: Anyone who likes to sweat, someone who wants a more physical practice, or those who like routine.

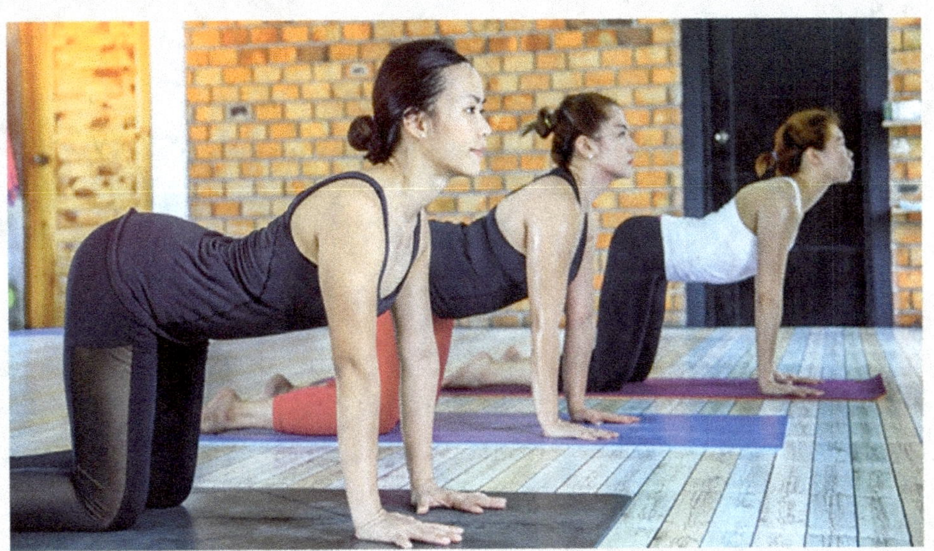

Power Yoga

Like vinyasa yoga, power yoga traces its roots to ashtanga but is less regimented and is more open to interpretation by individual teachers. "Power yoga is generally more active and is done at a quicker pace than other styles of yoga," says Chun.

Sleik adds that "power yoga strengthens the muscles while also increasing flexibility. The variation of sequences keeps the brain engaged while you work all muscle groups in the body."

Power yoga can be hot yoga or not, and some studios offer a mix of power and slow flow yoga to ease students into this intense practice. Fans of power yoga may also like buti yoga, which is just as physical but also includes tribal dance, primal movements, and plenty of core work.

Who Might Like It: Those who like ashtanga but want less rigidity, anyone who wants a good workout, and anyone who wants a less spiritual yoga practice.

Sivananda Yoga

Sivananda yoga is a form of hatha yoga based on the teachings of Hindu spiritual teacher Swami Sivananda. Classes are generally relaxing: while most yoga classes end with savasana (a final relaxation/corpse pose).

Sivananda starts with this pose, then moves into breathing exercises, sun salutations, and then 12 basic asanas.

Kearney likes this practice for "someone looking for more spiritual or energetic work," while Saunders says such Sivananda yoga can help push yourself to the next level if you're a beginner. Designed to support overall health and wellness, Sivananda yoga is appropriate for all levels and ages.

Who Might Like It: Those looking for a gentler form of yoga, anyone who wants a more spiritual practice.

Restorative Yoga

If you walked by a restorative yoga class, you might think everyone was taking a nap on their mats. This form of yoga uses props to support the body. The goal is to completely relax into poses, which are held for at least five minutes but often longer. This means that you might only do a handful of poses in a class, and it's perfectly acceptable to drift into sleep during them.

Some teachers might even lead you through yoga nidra – a guided meditation that allows you to hover blissfully between sleep and wake. One hour in yoga nidra is said to equal a few hours of shuteye, and while that can be a good self-care tool, it can't replace a healthy night's sleep.

Though all different types of yoga can aid stress relief and brain health, restorative yoga places its focus on down-regulating the nervous system. Restorative yoga can benefit those who need to chill out and de-stress, and it can also be used as part of your rest-day self-care. "Taking time to relax in a restorative class can have a huge impact on an athlete," says Kearney.

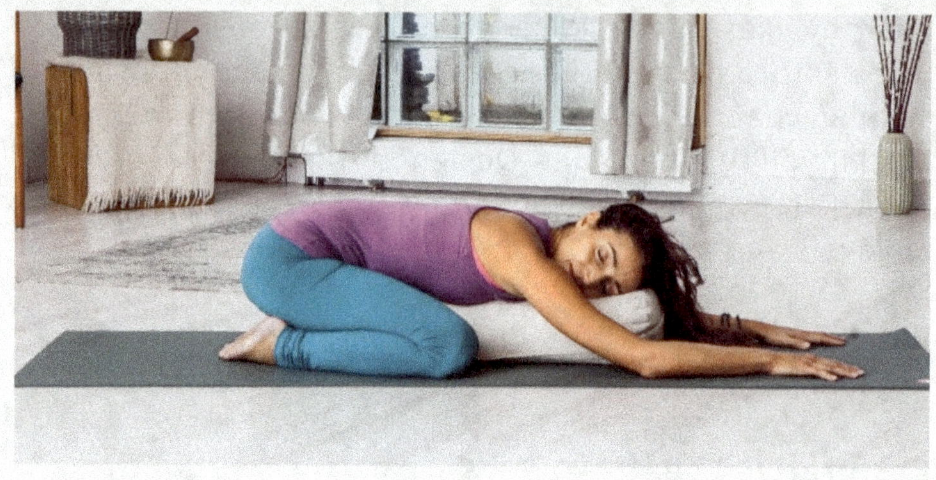

Who Might Like It: Anyone who needs to de-stress, those dealing with pain, and someone who struggles to relax.

Prenatal Yoga

Yoga can be a wonderful workout for moms-to-be. It often focuses on easing pains associated with pregnancy, such as sore hips or an aching low back. Prenatal yogaprovides stress relief, exercise, and self-care in one session, and the breathing exercises can come in handy during labor and delivery.

Since this is a practice designed specifically for moms-to-be, it excludes poses that might be too taxing or unsafe for the changing body. (But make sure you check in with your doctor before beginning a yoga practice, if you are pregnant.) Yoga for pregnancy, such as the Active Maternity series on Beachbody On Demand, also often includes plenty of exercises to prepare your body for delivery, like squats and pelvic floor work.

Who Might Like It: Moms-to-be and new moms who are easing back into exercise.

Aerial Yoga

Aerial yoga — sometimes called anti-gravity yoga — is relatively new, but quickly catching on. It involves traditional yoga poses with the added support of a strong, silky hammock that hangs from the ceiling. The hammock is used as a supportive prop in poses like pigeon or downward dog, and helps you more easily perform inverted poses (like headstands and handstands) that might be beyond your abilities or comfort levels. It's also used for a cocoon-like savasana (the final resting pose at the end of a yoga class). Classes can be either physically challenging or relaxing.

"Teaching aerial yoga has been so rewarding for me because I get to witness beginners gain body awareness and overcome fear of being inverted," says Melissa Vance, RYT (Registered Yoga Teacher) 200, an aerial yoga teacher based outside of Atlanta. "Hanging upside down reverses the blood flow in the body and decompresses the spine providing much relief and a euphoric feeling."

Who Might Like It: Those who want a nontraditional yoga experience, or anyone who wants the benefits of inversions but might fear going upside down on their own.

Acro yoga

Acro yoga takes familiar yoga poses — like downward dog or plank — and makes them double the fun (and sometimes double the work) by adding a partner. One partner serves as the "base" on the ground, while the other is the "flyer" who contorts themselves on the soles of the base's feet. (A spotter should always be involved for safety). "[Acro yoga] allows people to break from the rectangular confines of their yoga mat and find a connection with their fellow practitioners," says Lyle Mitchell, a YogaSlackers acro yoga teacher in Asheville, NC.

This type of yoga helps you playfully explore your mind-body connection, develops effective communication skills with a partner, and aids in setting appropriate boundaries. "Exploring these skills through acro yoga can translate to strengthening these skills in all our other relationships in life," he says. Saunders recommends acro yoga "if you are looking for the physical benefits of yoga in a fun and interactive environment." If you work as a base, it builds a strong lower body and core. Working as a flyer requires flexibility and strength, not to mention trust.

Who Might Like It: Those who enjoy practicing with a partner, couples looking to build trust and intimacy, or anyone with an adventurous streak who likes to go upside down.

YOGA FOR STRESS RELIEF

While stress is a common occurrence in life, living with stress for prolonged periods can affect a person's physical and mental health.

According to the American Psychological Association, the signs and symptoms of stress can include gastrointestinal difficulties, sleep problems, high blood pressure, fatigue, irritability, and cognitive concerns.

Yoga can help relax both the body and the mind and provide a wealth of benefits related to mental health.

Recent studies have shown a significant correlation between an active yoga practice and stress relief.

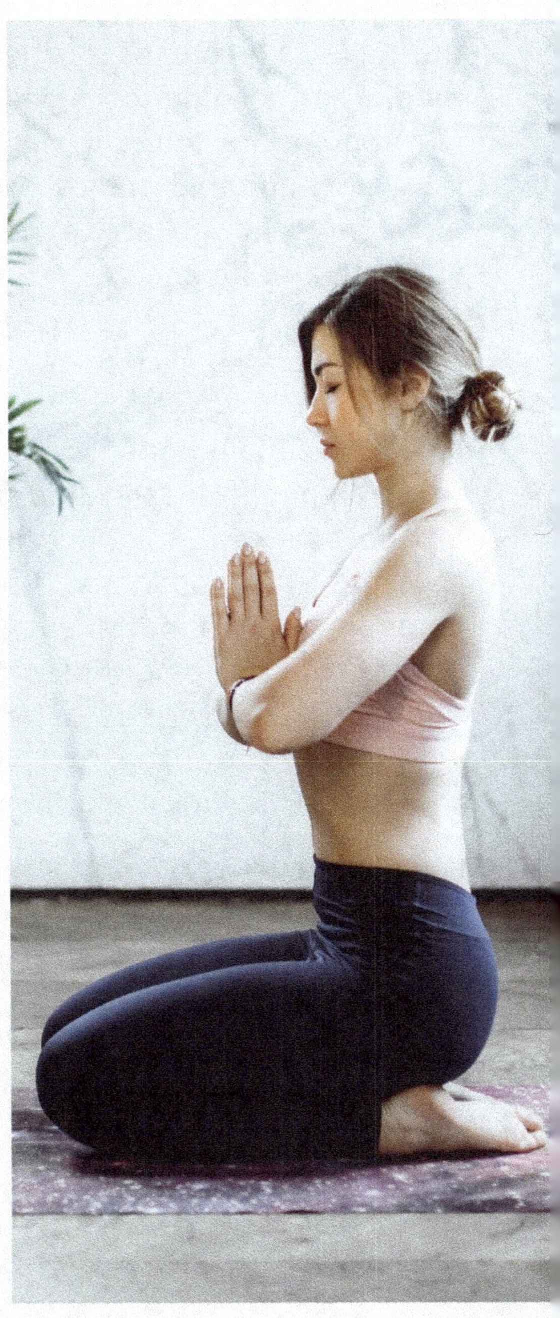

Yoga can help mitigate stress responses by controlling breathing and bodily movements, as well as by focusing the mind on physical experience rather than anxious thoughts. People often describe their mental state during yoga as one of clarity, calm, and focus. Like meditation techniques, a yoga practice can help to clear the mind of unwanted thoughts and encourage harmony between mind and body. Yoga can also serve as an effective form of exercise, helping you develop muscle strength and flexibility.

Mindfulness

One of the main benefits of yoga for stress relief is a focus on mindfulness. Mindfulness can help reduce anxiety as it centers on a calm, observant focus on your thoughts and sensations. One of the common components of mindfulness tends to be an observance of thoughts and emotions without judgment. Instead, mindfulness allows you to be fully present and in tune with the sensations of your body along with any thoughts or feelings that might arise.

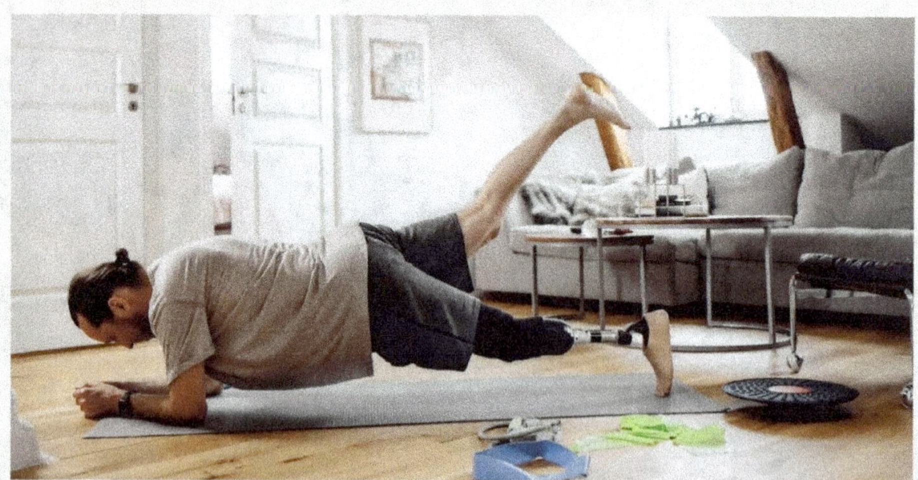

Meditation

Meditation is a practice that often includes mindfulness, and it can be cultivated during a yoga practice. Meditation is a core component of some Eastern religious practices, and it has been a part of some forms of yoga for centuries. Meditation has been shown to help reduce anxiety, including symptoms like excessive stress, panic, and agoraphobia. Some research shows that meditation can even help reduce your blood pressure and mitigate insomnia. The quiet, rhythmic movements of yoga may help to induce a meditative state, while a focus on breathing can promote a sense of calm.

As with mindfulness, one of the core components of meditation is often an acceptance of whatever you are experiencing in the moment. Instead of dwelling on your stress or anxiety, you can acknowledge it and let it pass through you without letting it consume you.

Exercise

Yoga, which focuses on movements as well as stretching and flexibility, can be an effective way to exercise and stay fit. Exercise has also been shown to be effective in fighting symptoms of anxiety. Exercise helps promote both mental and physical health as it releases endorphins, a feel-good chemical that helps promote mental health.

Exercise can also help to occupy your mind and distract you from negative thoughts and feelings.

Even a few minutes of exercise a day or a simple 20-minute yoga routine may be enough to reap the mental and physical benefits of exercise.

Stretching

Since muscle tension and soreness can be common symptoms of stress and anxiety, people experiencing these concerns tend to experience tightness and pain throughout their bodies. Yoga may directly address and resolve anxiety symptoms that manifest as soreness and tension. Yoga works to stretch out the muscles, gently flowing through motions that elongate and exercise muscles throughout the body.

Whether you find your shoulders aching at the end of a stressful day, or you feel physically exhausted from managing stress, yoga can serve as a gentle way of increasing your awareness of your physical self and relieving tension throughout your body.

Spiritual effects

While many people may consider yoga a form of exercise rather than a spiritual activity, yoga has its roots as a spiritual practice that helps to unify the mind and body.

Yoga teaches practitioners to focus on mindfulness and to calmly accept thoughts, feelings, and sensations as they occur. For some, one of the goals of yoga is spiritual enlightenment. In this respect, a spiritual yoga practice can be aligned with improved mental health.

Even if you are not sure what yoga might mean to you in terms of spirituality, it can be an effective way to delve deeper into yourself and find a sense of inner calm in the process.

Yoga for beginners

If you're interested in yoga but aren't sure where to start, you might consider attending a beginner's yoga class at a local gym or fitness center. There are usually affordable (or even free) yoga options for beginners, as well as classes with individual instruction. If you are not sure what style you want to focus on, consider attending a wide range of classes to determine what works best for you. Also, you might speak with a yoga instructor about their own practice. Many yoga instructors are happy to assist someone new to yoga in learning more about the practice.

Seeking help for stress

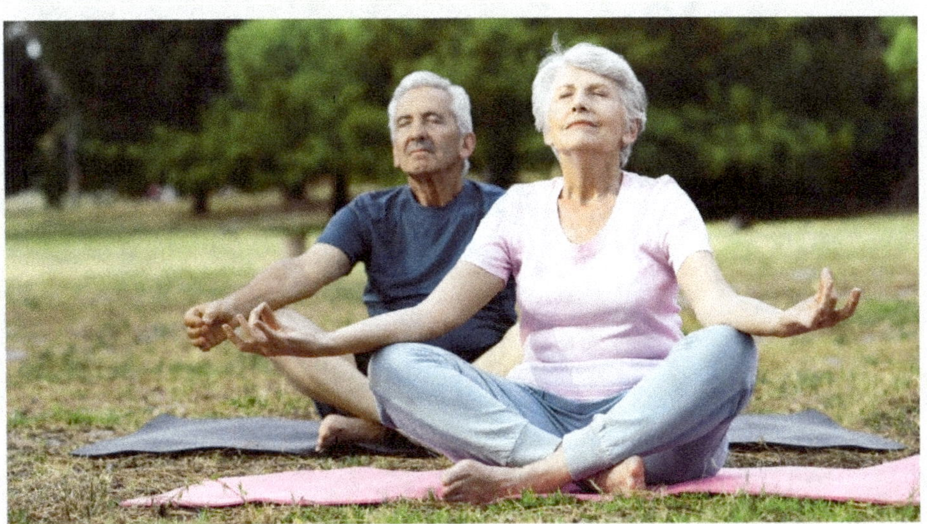

Stress can have a major impact on a person's health and well-being, both physically and emotionally. It can intensify emotions (such as fear) and may cause you to stop doing things that you once enjoyed.

Stress disorders can also have an impact on personal relationships, your ability to work effectively, and your ability to form new relationships. If you are concerned you have a stress disorder, consider speaking with a mental health professional.

In therapy, you might learn to identify what is causing your stress and learn several new coping strategies. Additionally, a therapist may be able to help you build strategies that promote resilience to manage current and future stressful events.

How does Yoga Reduce
Stress and anxiety

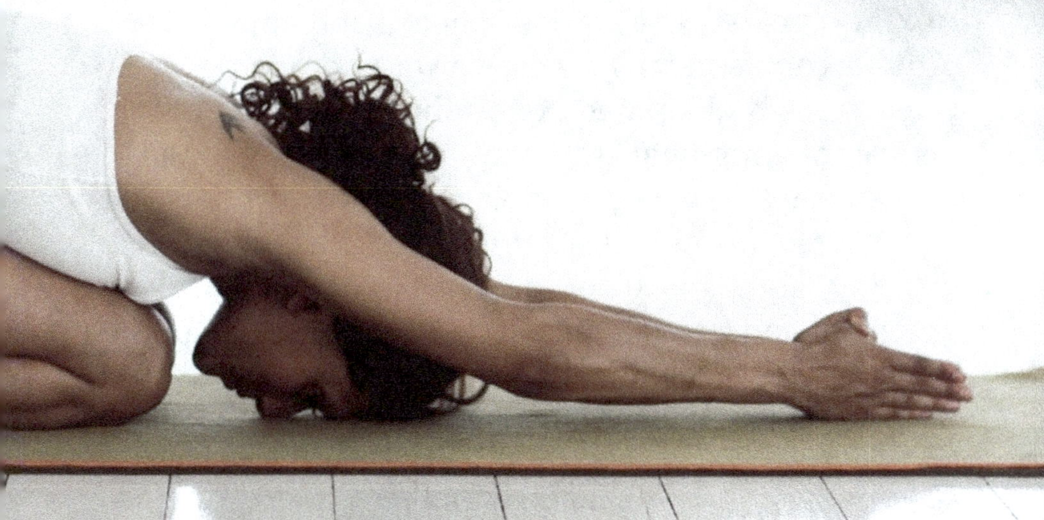

UNDERSTANDING STRESS AND ANXIETY

Stress: Stress is the body's natural response to a perceived threat, challenge, or demand. It's a physiological and psychological reaction that prepares an individual to cope with a situation. In a stress response, the body releases hormones like cortisol and adrenaline, which increase alertness and energy. Stress can be triggered by various factors, including work deadlines, financial pressures, personal relationships, and more. While acute stress can be beneficial, chronic stress, which persists over an extended period, can have adverse effects on mental and physical health.

Anxiety: Anxiety is a state of unease and apprehension, often accompanied by excessive worry or fear, even when there is no immediate or obvious threat. It is a persistent emotional state that can range from mild uneasiness to severe panic. Anxiety disorders, such as generalized anxiety disorder (GAD), social anxiety disorder, and panic disorder, are characterized by excessive and irrational anxiety. These conditions can interfere with daily life and well-being. Anxiety often involves cognitive, emotional, and physical symptoms, and it can manifest in various ways, including restlessness, rapid heartbeat, and irrational fears.

In summary, stress is a natural response to a perceived threat or challenge, while anxiety represents a more prolonged and often irrational state of unease and apprehension.

Both stress and anxiety can have significant impacts on an individual's mental and physical health, making them important subjects to address in the context of well-being and stress reduction techniques like yoga.

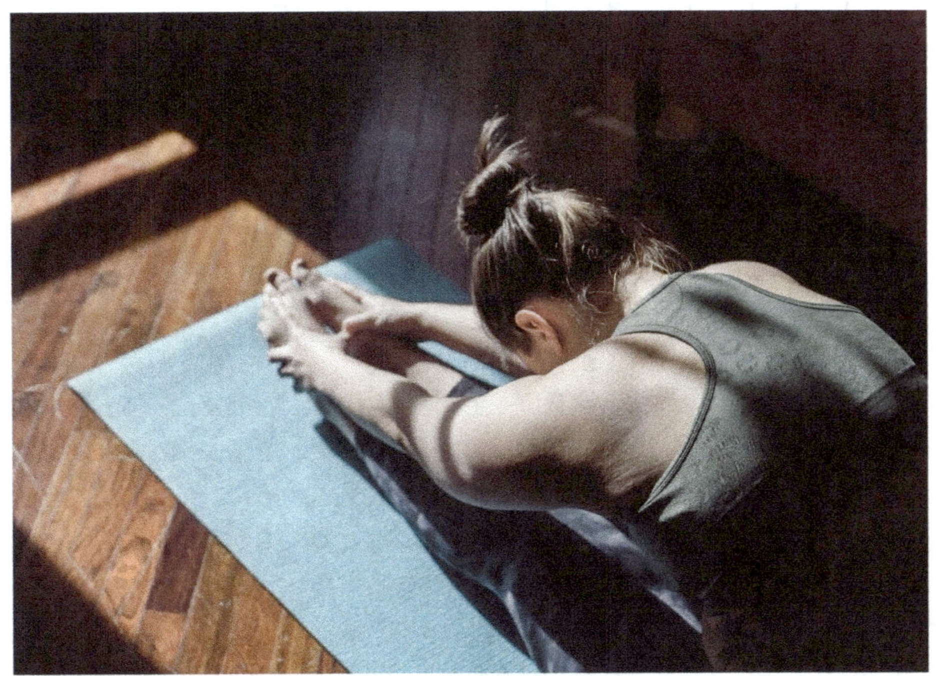

CAUSES OF STRESS AND ANXIETY

Stress and anxiety can stem from a variety of sources and triggers. Understanding these causes is essential to effectively address and manage these conditions.

Here are some common causes:

1. Work-Related Stress: Job pressures, deadlines, long working hours, and the fear of job loss can lead to stress and anxiety. Workplace stress is a significant contributor to these conditions.
2. Financial Concerns: Worries about money, debt, and financial instability can be a major source of stress and anxiety for many individuals and families.
3. Relationship Issues: Conflicts in personal relationships, including romantic relationships, family dynamics, and friendships, can result in emotional distress.
4. Health Concerns: Dealing with chronic illnesses, medical conditions, or the health of a loved one can be extremely stressful. Health-related anxiety can also manifest in the fear of illness or hypochondria.
5. Major Life Changes: Significant life events such as marriage, divorce, parenthood, relocation, or the loss of a loved one can trigger stress and anxiety due to the adjustments and uncertainties they bring.
6. Academic Pressure: Students often experience stress and anxiety due to academic expectations, exams, and the pressure to excel in their studies.
7. Traumatic Events: Experiencing or witnessing traumatic events, such as accidents or natural disasters, can lead to post-traumatic stress disorder (PTSD) and ongoing anxiety.
8. Social Pressures: Societal expectations, cultural norms, and the pressure to conform to certain standards can create stress, particularly for individuals who feel they don't meet these expectations.

9. Environmental Factors: Living in noisy or polluted environments can contribute to stress. Lack of access to green spaces and nature can also be a stressor.
10. Information Overload: Constant exposure to news, social media, and technology can lead to information overload, contributing to feelings of overwhelm and anxiety.
11. Genetics and Biology: Genetic predisposition and imbalances in brain chemistry can make some individuals more susceptible to anxiety disorders.
12. Substance Abuse: The use of alcohol, drugs, or other substances to cope with stress or anxiety can lead to a vicious cycle of addiction and worsening mental health.

Recognizing the diverse causes of stress and anxiety highlights the need for individualized approaches to coping and treatment. It's important to address the specific sources of stress and anxiety in one's life when seeking ways to manage and alleviate these conditions effectively.

HOW STRESS AND ANXIETY AFFECTS HEALTH?

Stress and anxiety can have profound effects on both mental and physical health. These conditions, when left unmanaged, can lead to a wide range of health issues. Here's an overview of how stress and anxiety affect health:

1. Mental Health Disorders: Prolonged stress and anxiety can contribute to the development or exacerbation of mental health disorders such as depression, generalized anxiety disorder, panic disorder, and post-traumatic stress disorder (PTSD).
2. Cardiovascular Problems: Chronic stress can increase the risk of heart disease, high blood pressure, and atherosclerosis (hardening of the arteries), which can lead to heart attacks and strokes.
3. Immune System Suppression: Stress and anxiety can weaken the immune system's ability to fight off infections and illnesses, making individuals more susceptible to colds, flu, and other diseases.
4. Gastrointestinal Issues: These conditions can lead to digestive problems, including irritable bowel syndrome (IBS), indigestion, and stomach ulcers.
5. Sleep Disturbances: Stress and anxiety often result in sleep difficulties, including insomnia, which can, in turn, lead to a range of health problems, including reduced cognitive function and an increased risk of accidents.

6. Weight Fluctuations: Stress can lead to overeating or undereating, which can result in weight gain or loss. These fluctuations can contribute to obesity or malnutrition.
7. Muscle Tension and Pain: Stress and anxiety can cause muscle tension, leading to conditions like tension headaches, migraines, and temporomandibular joint disorder (TMJ).
8. Respiratory Issues: Individuals experiencing anxiety may have shallow breathing or hyperventilation, which can exacerbate respiratory conditions such as asthma.
9. Skin Problems: Stress and anxiety can lead to skin conditions such as eczema, psoriasis, and acne.
10. Cognitive Impairment: Persistent stress and anxiety can impair cognitive function, including memory and concentration.
11. Behavioral Issues: People under chronic stress may resort to unhealthy coping mechanisms like substance abuse, overeating, or self-isolation, which can further compound their health problems.
12. Hormonal Imbalances: Stress can disrupt hormonal balance, leading to issues like irregular menstrual cycles in women and reduced fertility
13. Weakened Coping Abilities: Constant stress and anxiety can erode an individual's ability to cope with life's challenges, leading to a cycle of escalating stress and mental health issues.

Understanding the profound impact of stress and anxiety on health underscores the importance of proactive stress management and the use of techniques like yoga to mitigate these effects. It also highlights the need for seeking professional help when necessary to address mental health concerns.

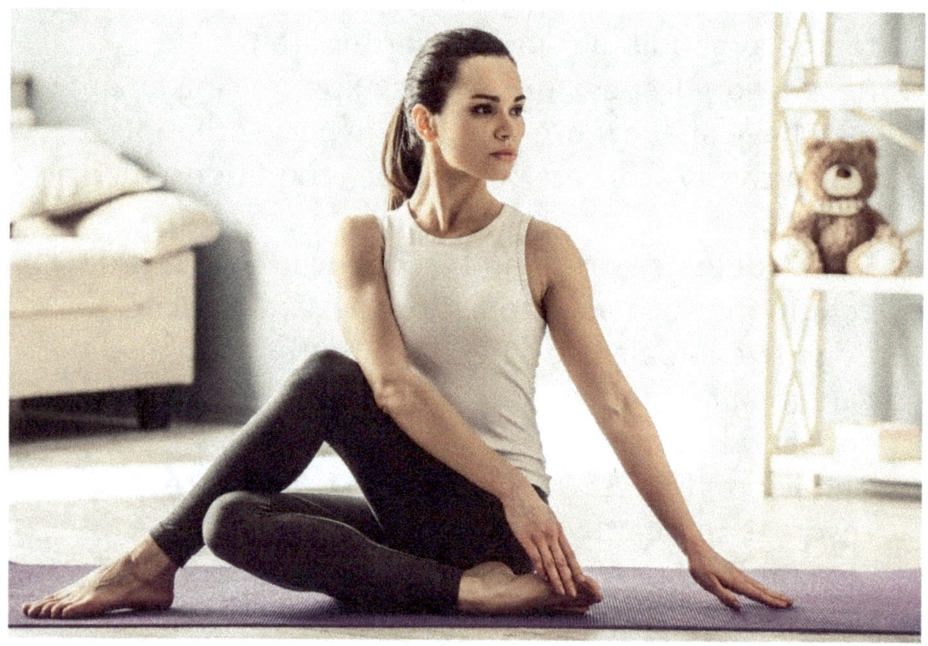

Prepare Before Your Yoga

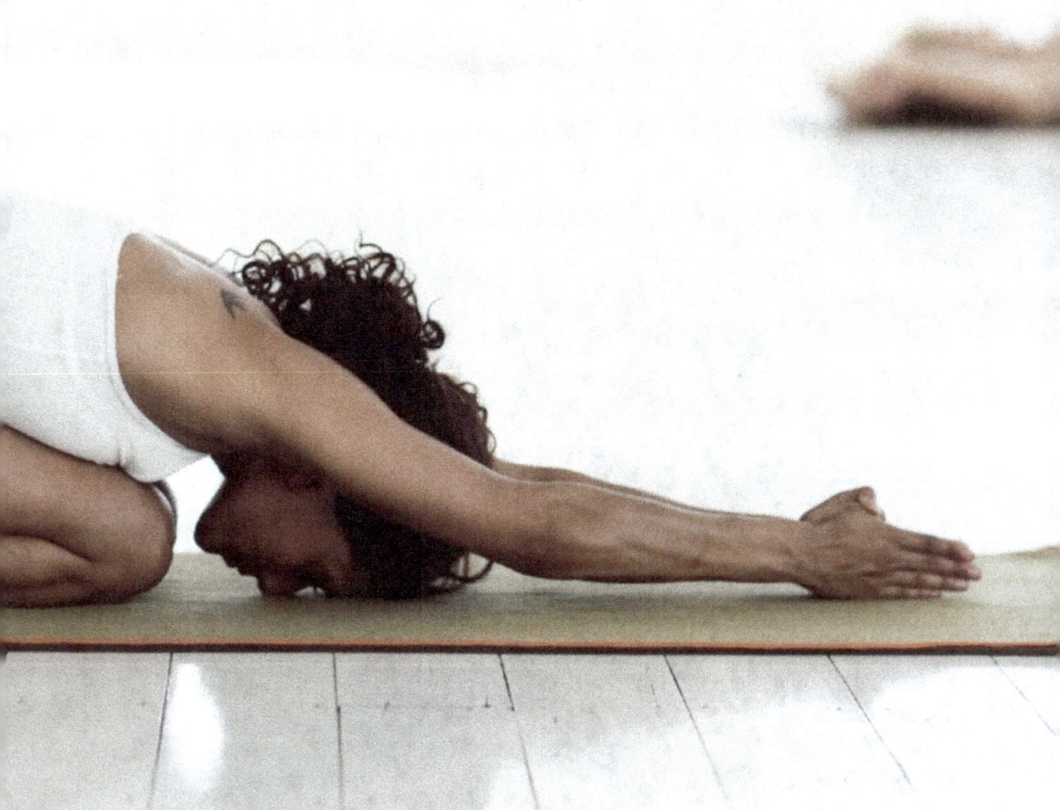

WHAT TO WEAR

While it may seem like you need to get decked out in designer yoga gear before you head to class, that couldn't be farther from the truth. For your first few classes, wear items you already have on hand, and keep things as simple as possible. Here are a few tips:

Shoes

Yoga is most often done barefoot. You will occasionally see people with some kind of sock or shoe, but that's often due to an injury or medical condition. If you feel completely uncomfortable taking off your shoes in front of strangers, compromise by wearing yoga socks. These special socks have non-slip grips on the bottom that "grab" the mat and prevent your feet from slipping around.

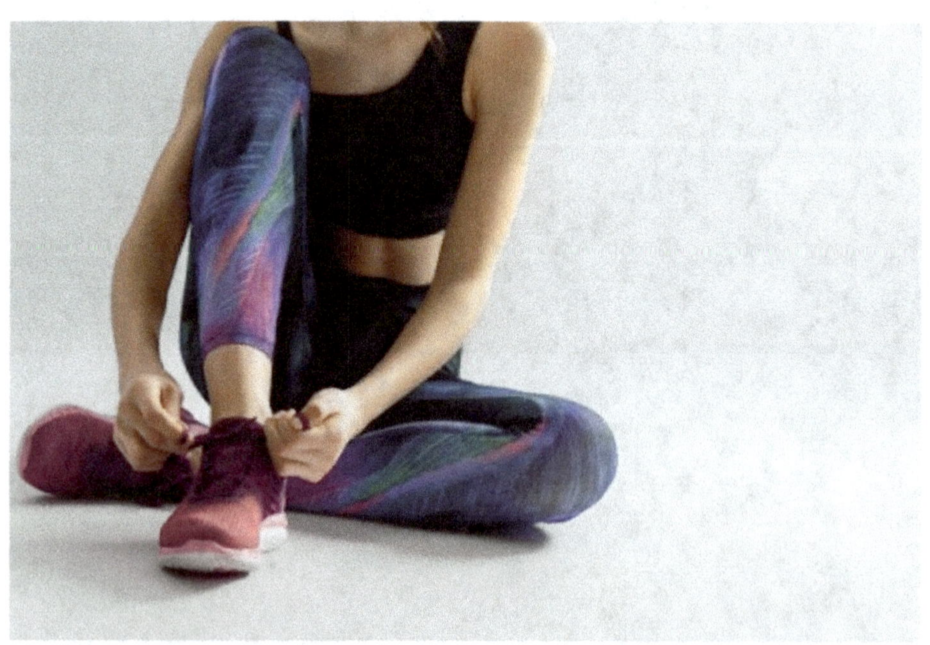

Pants

There are many different styles of yoga pants for women and men, but you don't have to run out and buy a special pair before your very first class. Any comfortable exercise pants or shorts will do, just make sure you avoid pants that don't stretch, like jeans.

After a few classes, you may decide you need pants that are shorter, longer, looser, higher-waisted, or not falling every time you stretch up. That's a good time to go shopping. You can stick to big box stores like Target or Walmart, both of which have athletic apparel lines, or you can seek out specialty retailers geared specifically to the yoga market—wear your favorite pair of Alo leggings, for example. Although it is based on personal preference and the type of yoga you are doing, yoga pants and shorts for men often have a looser fit, while women often prefer form-fitting spandex or Lycra-blend legging.

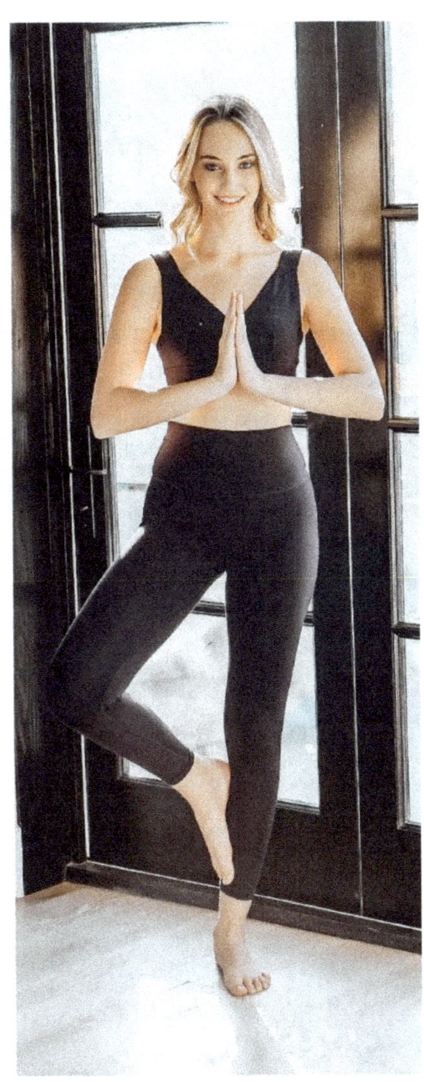

Tops

A shirt that's a little bit fitted works best for yoga. Big baggy t-shirts, or even loose-fitting workout shirts, aren't great since they'll slide down every time you bend over...and you're going to be doing a lot of bending over. Sleeveless tops are popular since they allow freedom of movement in the arms and shoulders. Wear whatever kind of bra you prefer for exercising.

EQUIPMENTS FOR YOGA

One of the great things about yoga is that you don't need tons of yoga equipment and accessories in order to be successful. Equipment for yoga is simply used to extend your skill level and to offer your body that extra support when needed.

When questioning "what yoga equipment do I need for yoga?" you should take into consideration that some of the most basic yoga equipment that will feature on this list is a necessity to your practice. These basic yoga equipment pieces are:

Yoga Mat
Yoga Mat Bag
Comfortable Exercise Clothes
Water Bottle
Yoga Block
Yoga Strap

However, whilst other pieces of yoga exercise equipment are not vital to your practice, they will allow you to challenge and push yourself in specific areas, such as aerial yoga. For this reason, we have decided to cover a wide variety of products, in order to ensure that there is something for everyone and not just beginners interested in the basics.

While this is both an advanced and beginner's guide to yoga equipment and accessories, it is important to realise that one size does not fit all.

Many of you who are reading this may be looking to buy the basics, in order to practice vinyasa or hatha yoga. Alternatively, some of you may be reading this wanting to explore a niche type of yoga, such as aerial, and will be looking to buy yoga fitness equipment that will assist in that area.

1. Yoga Mat

Regardless of whether you're using your own or yoga studio equipment, you need a yoga mat in order to practice yoga. There is no way around this fact, the yoga mat is the most vital piece of yoga exercise equipment.

If you purchase just one thing on this list today, buy yourself a yoga mat.

In terms of equipment for yoga, the mats will benefit you when practicing as they offer more grip than any kind of flooring. Nobody wants to injure themselves when exercising, which is why it is so important to buy yoga equipment that will keep us safe.

Not only will yoga mats offer your hands and feet more grip when entering poses and holds, but they will also cushion your fall in the worst-case scenarios of slipping or tumbling.

Another benefit of purchasing this piece of equipment is now more prevalent than ever in the age of Covid. Yoga mats are also really easy to clean, so if you're returning to the yoga studio for the first time post-lockdown you can put all health and safety worries to ease.

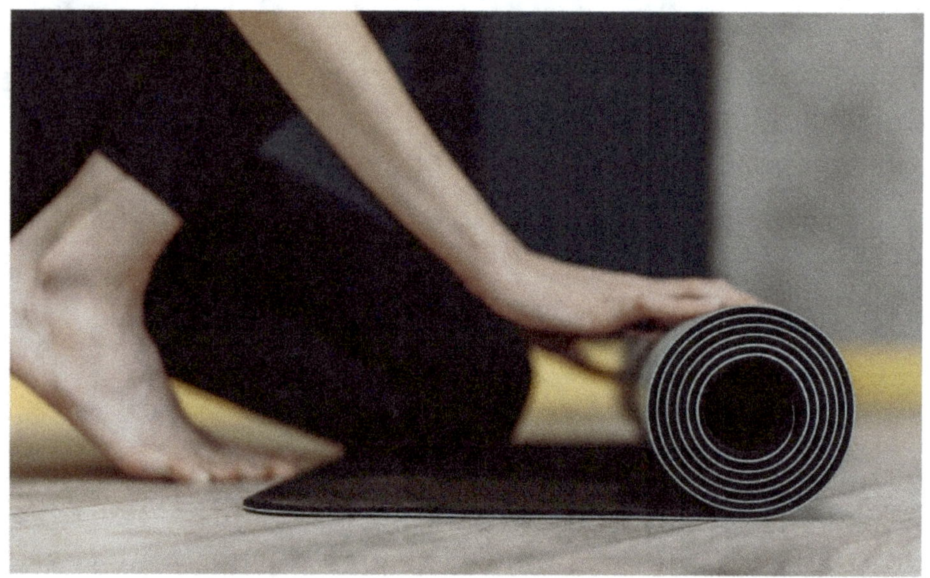

2. Yoga Mat Bag

When looking at yoga equipment for beginners, one of the most often overlooked pieces of equipment is the yoga mat bag. If you're practising yoga solely from home this may not seem 'vital', but if you're looking to join a class, then you're going to want to carry your equipment in the most efficient way possible.

Most gym bags, backpacks and handbags simply don't have room to accommodate the unique shape and size of yoga mats. You don't want to be squishing your mat into a bag, and potentially damaging it in the process.

This is why the yoga mat bag is such an essential purchase when you buy yoga equipment.

So, instead of either coming to class flustered and struggling to carry everything you need or potentially breaking your expensive equipment by forcing it into a gym bag, we would recommend simply buying a yoga mat bag. It is a smart investment in the long run that will save you money in not having to replace broken or damaged equipment.

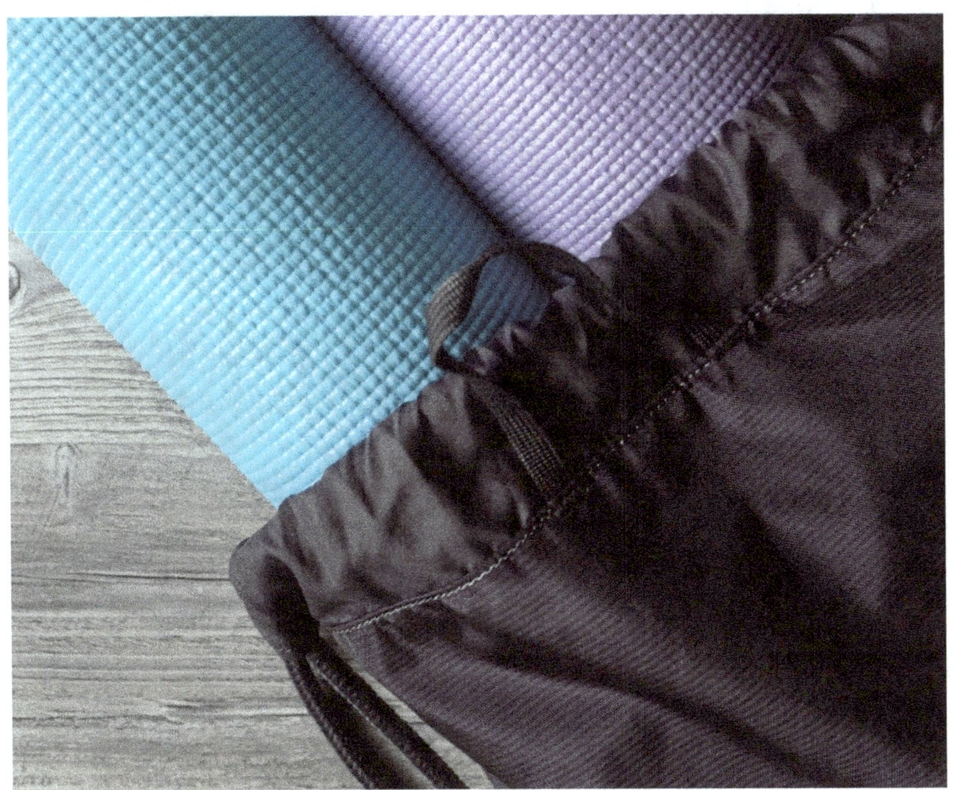

3. Yoga Towels

If yoga mats are viewed as basic yoga equipment, then consider yoga towels the Bikram yoga equipment equivalent.

The rise of Bikram yoga, or as it is otherwise known as 'hot yoga', has birthed a new wave of yoga fitness equipment. For those of you who want to get into hot yoga, consider the yoga towel to be the most vital piece of Bikram yoga equipment you can own.

But what is a yoga towel and what does it do?

When practicing hot yoga you're obviously going to sweat more (that is the whole purpose of the class after all!). But what the sweat can do is actually make the mat dangerous for you to use, as well as making it more likely to slip or move on the floor.

The yoga towel can be placed on top of the mat and prevents it from becoming slippery with sweat. An advantage of using the mat is that the more you sweat the more grip it will have, the towel will absorb the sweat and create resistance against the mat and floor.

The yoga towel is a specially designed piece of Bikram yoga equipment as regular towels will not provide the same type of support.

Additionally, if you sweat a lot and are worried about the towel becoming slippery and losing grip, we'd recommend looking for towels with non-slip backings, such as ones that come with silicone nubs. Not only is this a great piece of Bikram yoga equipment, but it can also be placed on top of yoga mats during regular yoga classes, should you want to avoid any dirty/pre-used mats.

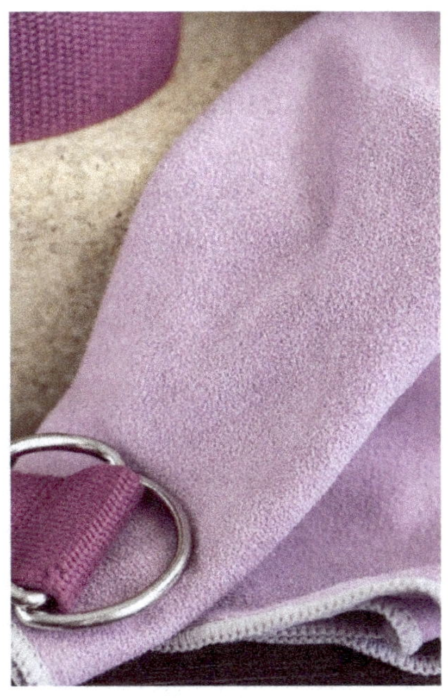

4. Water Bottles

It's so important to stay hydrated when exercising, and often many newbie yogis forget the fact that yoga is an intense workout. You wouldn't practice without a mat, and you should take that same kind of energy when it comes to bringing a water bottle to the studio/class with you.

Treat your water bottle as a piece of equipment that is needed for yoga, not an optional accessory, similar to the need for running water bottles during running! The more water we lose from sweating, the more water we have to replace through drinking. If the average person weighs 150 pounds, then that means their body consists of 5 litres of water.

5. Yoga Straps

Yoga straps are pieces of equipment that are used in yoga to assist in the development of flexibility. If you're a beginner with no previous flexibility training, then we would recommend investing in some yoga straps as they will decrease the likelihood of muscle straining.

You don't even need to use the straps in crazy elaborate poses, you will see and feel the benefit that yoga straps can provide from even the simplest of movements, such as sitting poses that use the yoga strap to stretch your legs.

One commonly used technique of this yoga apparatus is to grab both ends of the strap and pull it towards you whilst leaning into a pose.

So if we use the example of the pose mentioned above, we would be wrapping the strap around our feet and pulling them either towards our back or chest as we enter the pose. However, the strap is a multipurpose piece of yoga equipment and can also be used on the buttocks, knees and hips too.

The poses and stretches that are used with the strap can effectively decrease tension whilst increasing flexibility. To increase flexibility along with your balance, we would recommend using the strap in the upright position.

6. Yoga Wheel

The next entry onto our yoga equipment list is relatively new with it becoming a popular piece of yoga studio equipment in 2018.

The yoga wheel is a hollow, circular-shaped prop that is similar to the yoga block, in the sense that is designed to aid in stretching, releasing tension and improving your flexibility.

As previously mentioned the yoga wheel has similar benefits to that of the yoga block. It will help to improve your flexibility, by adding extra support for your limbs, however, because it rolls it will allow you to stretch your body even further.

Additionally, the yoga wheel is a great piece of equipment for yoga as you'll be able to stretch back and forth, whilst also allowing yourself to get into deeper positions.

Now that we have covered how the yoga wheel and yoga block are similar, we must mention the unique benefits that the yoga wheel poses. If you suffer from any back pains or spinal issues, you can use the yoga wheel to ease this pain.

Simply lie on top of the wheel and begin to push your body back and forth, paying particular attention to the areas where you feel the most pain.

The yoga wheel is also a good piece of equipment used in yoga wind-down sessions and is great for relaxing tense muscles.

If you're having trouble sleeping after a nightly exercise, we would recommend switching to yoga wheel assisted practices for a night of better sleep.

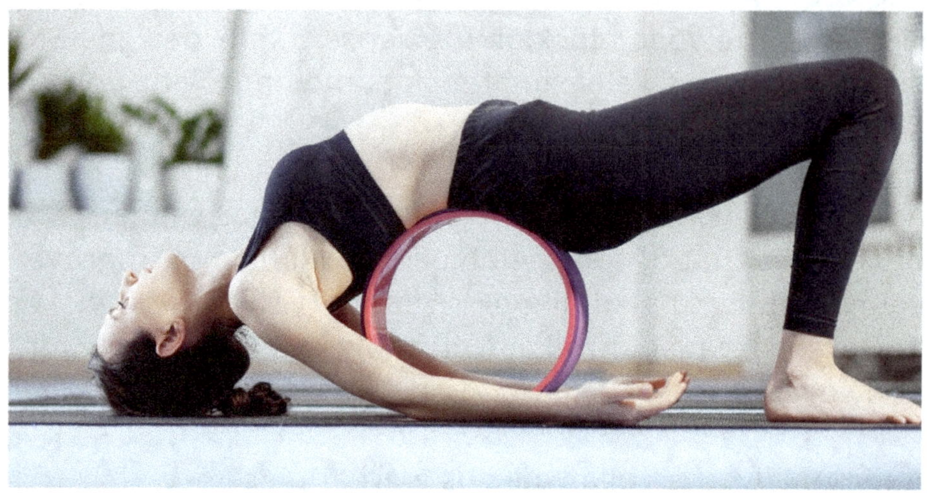

7. Massage Guns

Whilst we're on the topic of the best yoga equipment for post-workout routines, we would recommend purchasing a massage gun.

When purchasing yoga equipment for beginners, you may have a tendency to just buy products that will help you during the yoga class or session itself. But it's also important to invest in products that will help your body once the class is over.

Compared to a lot of the entries on this list, this will be more of a pricey purchase, but consider it portable therapy for your muscles.

Massage guns will relax your muscles after a tiring workout or stretching session. Many of these massage guns will treat your muscles with percussion therapy, which can make you happy by releasing serotonin in your body. This will put your mind at ease and make you a happier person.

The foam roller and yoga wheel can stay to one side, because this advanced yoga apparatus will ease tension within your muscles and joints, by stimulating the blood flow to these areas.

Increased blood flow can not only ease joint aches and pains but can also promote a faster metabolism, which in turn can translate to weight loss, healthier bowels and a better sleeping pattern.

Additionally, we would recommend using the gun for 15-20 minutes following a stressful workday: especially if you're someone who is hunched over a computer all day, the massage gun can greatly ease any pains and aches your desk chair may cause.

8. Meditation Pillow

If you're someone who wants to get into meditation but struggles to stay comfortable on a hardwood floor, we would recommend investing in a meditation pillow. Couch cushions are fine, but meditation pillows are some of the most overlooked pieces of equipment used in yoga.

Specially designed to hold your body up tall as you sit cross-legged on the ground, the meditation pillows are comfortable and will help to align your spine into its correct curvature. Sitting flat on the ground or on a regular pillow will not provide your body with this level of support, in fact, doing so can even damage the range of motion in your hips. However, the meditation pillow does support your hips and once you sit down on it, the pillow will help to move your hips forward slightly, in order to align with the curvature of your back. Meditation pillows are traditionally round but have evolved over time to compensate for different individuals' needs. Some are crescent-shaped which are designed specifically to support your thighs. It is important to note, however, that if you purchase meditation pillows of this shape tuck your ankles in towards your body to keep them off the floor.

Regardless of what kind of pillow you choose to purchase, if you feel discomfort in your ankles we would recommend placing the mediation pillow on top of a blanket. That way not only does your body have extra support but you'll be completely comfortable whilst doing it. Remember mediation is all about relaxation: being comfortable during this process should be your top priority.

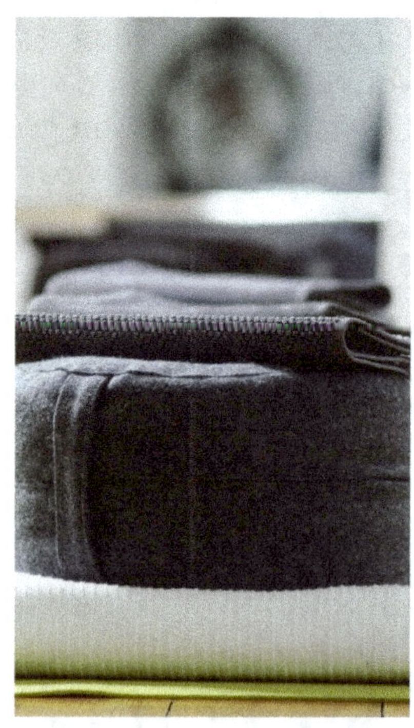

9. Eye Pillows

Also used in restorative yoga are eye pillows, which look very similar to sandbags but function slightly differently.

The eye pillow is obviously placed over your eyes during meditation or restorative yoga sessions, with one of its main benefits being the regulation of your nervous system, mood, digestion and even the immune system.

Traditionally, yoga eye pillows are filled with flax seeds. Once it's on your face, the lightweight contents combined with the soft textured fabric will penetrate the vagus nerve.

This nerve represents the main component of the parasympathetic nervous system, which oversees everything from the previously mentioned mood, digestion and immune system.

This nerve essentially establishes a connection between the brain and the rest of the body, and once light pressure is applied to it, the vagus nerve will send a message to the rest of your body that it's in a state of peace. Relaxation can also be achieved through the perfect amount of pressure applied to your eyes, which will relax the muscles in the rest of your face and shoulders as a result too.

10. Yoga Chairs

Yoga can be misinterpreted by a lot of people as many think in order to achieve success in the practice you need to be a contortionist, but that simply isn't true.

If you struggle with mobility then yoga chairs can allow you to join in on the practice whilst doing so in a manner that is safe and comfortable for you.

In the same way that your body moves and flows through poses during traditional cycles of yoga, it can do so during chair yoga classes too. Any form of traditional yoga can be taught whilst using the yoga chair, it does not limit any possibility of learning the form you wish to pursue.

Without ever leaving the seat you can take advantage of the many benefits this yoga apparatus offers.

Using the yoga chair can help to improve your flexibility: remember flexibility is not gained from doing crazy elaborate poses and holds, flexibility is gained from extending your range of motion.

It is entirely unique to you and your body so take things as slow and gentle as you need to and you'll find the success you're looking for.

11. Posters And Pictures

Posters and pictures are surprisingly valuable accessories that any yogi can learn a lot from. Whether you choose to get posters that teach you poses, or are looking to simply decorate your home studio with some yoga symbols, posters and pictures can actually impart hundreds of years worth of knowledge.

Originally created by Indian mystics, yoga symbols were often used as a wordless form of communication. The creators of many symbols wanted their wisdom to transcend culture and language barriers, with the desire of imparting their teachings through a simple picture.

If you're interested in meditation we'd recommend getting a poster of a Mandala symbol. This symbol has calming properties, which can be activated by following its unique shapes and patterns with your eyes.

Similarly, posters that teach you poses also impart wisdom, and much like the online yoga classes will allow you to learn at your own rate.

Alternatively, you can use the posters to become better acquainted with the names of yoga poses. It's one thing to follow along with a class or video, it's a whole other thing to actively try to learn more about the practice.

12. Power Plate/Vibration Plates

Many of you may be familiar with power plates or vibration plates, but did you know that they can also be incorporated as yoga equipment too.

For those of you who aren't familiar with this equipment, power plates are exercise machines that you stand on top of, and they then send high-frequency vibrations through the muscles in your body. In terms of operating as yoga apparatus, many yogis love to use the power plates as structures to hold their poses on.

The most commonly sought after benefit of using power plates is weight loss. Due to the high-frequency vibrations, your metabolism actually increases in speed. However, simply participating in vibration yoga alone won't be enough to lose significant amounts of weight: for optimum results, we recommend pairing it with a balanced diet and plenty of water.

As we have already discussed, there are many kinds of yoga that will help tone the muscles in your body. However, if you're looking for significant toning, we would recommend trying vibration yoga as vibration plates alone have been proven to increase muscle toning, so pairing them with a practice such as yoga will result in your desired outcome.

Yoga Poses for Stress Relief

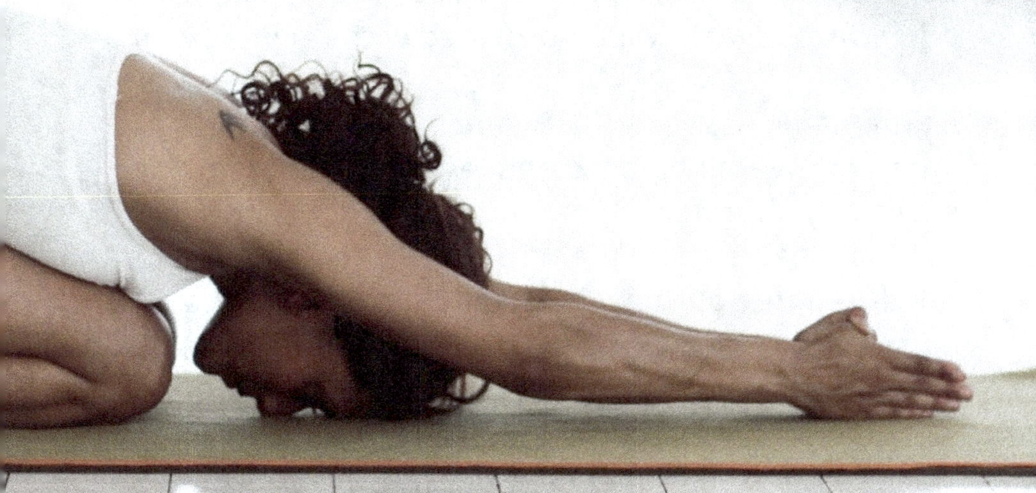

STICK POSE

Benefits & Purposes

The balancing stick pose is relatively simple to execute even for a beginner, though it does come with its fair share of benefits, the most notable of which being a tremendous relief of any stress and tension along your entire spine. Your body posture will improve as well, since the muscles of your lower back and shoulders will be strengthened.
You're entire circulatory system, and particularly the blood vessels in the heart itself, will be getting a tremendous workout as well, largely due to the horizontal alignment that your body will be in if you perform this posture properly. Your liver, spleen, and other vital organs will be provided with relief as well.

As the name suggest, the Balancing Stick posture improves overall balance and, as with all Bikram Yoga exercises, improves mental focus and concentration, as you will need a lot of them to sustain the position for the full duration. Your lower legs and particularly the inner muscles of your quadriceps (front of the thigh) will become stronger and will develop higher endurance.

Finally, and as a direct result of all of the above, the Balancing Stick posture will help you prevent (to an extent) heart-related diseases and conditions.

Directions

As you can see, the pose is fairly simple and does not require incredible flexibility, such as the Dandayamana Janushirasana for example. It does, however, require a great deal of balancing. Follow these steps exactly as laid out:

- Start by lifting your arms above your head and pointing them towards the ceiling. Your arm muscles should be kept tight and your elbows locked. Interlock all your fingers while making sure to keep your index fingers pointed outwards, just like if you were pretending your hands were a gun!

- Arch your lower back slightly while pushing your hips forward.
- Take a big step forward with your right leg, immediately locking it at the knee as soon as it touches the ground (the left leg remains back in place).

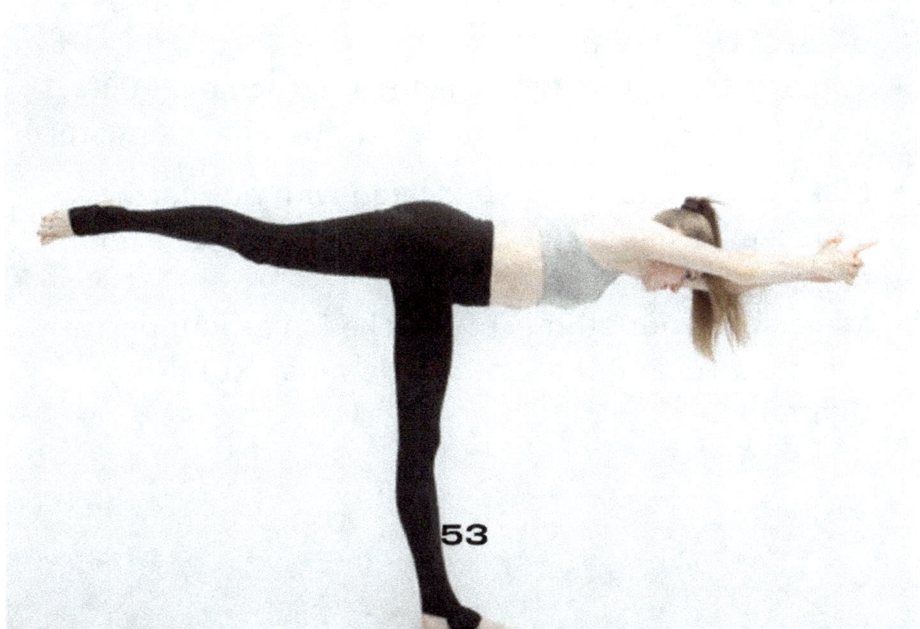

- Using your left leg as a pivot point, lower your upper body forward while simultaneously lifting up your left leg. This movement must be performed very quickly (one second at most) as you want the blood to come rushing to your head.
- At this point, your raised (left) leg, upper body and arms should all form a line that is perfectly parallel to the floor. If someone were to look at you from the side, you would look like the perfect letter T.
- Keep the foot of your supporting leg pointed perfectly forward, in the same direction your arms are pointing.
- Begin to stretch your body in two opposite directions – pull back with your lifted leg, and push forward with your torso and arms. While you do that, do not forget to maintain the perfect T-letter shape.
- Hold for 15 or so seconds or however long your instructor specifies, then lower your log and repeat the same procedure for the other leg.

Things to Keep in Mind

- Do not tuck your chin to your chest; keep your face parallel with the floor.
- You arms and supporting leg should remain 100% locked throughout the entire duration of the posture.

- Make sure to squeeze your head with both arms; squeeze hard, but not hard enough that your temples or ears start to hurt!
- Make sure your stomach is sucked in as you perform the posture, and that your abdominal muscles are tightened.

CORPSE POSE

Benefits & Purposes

Savasana allows your body and mind time to process what has happened during a yoga class, helping you wind down and relax. For this reason it is most often practiced at the end of a yoga session. It provides a necessary counterpoint to the effort you put forth during asana practice. You may also practice Savasana at home before sleeping as a way to quiet your mind and get more restful sleep.

Directions

Lie down on your back.

- Separate your legs. Let go of holding your legs straight so that your feet can fall open to either side.
- Bring your arms alongside your body, but slightly separated from your torso. Turn your palms to face upwards but don't try to keep them open. Let the fingers curl in.

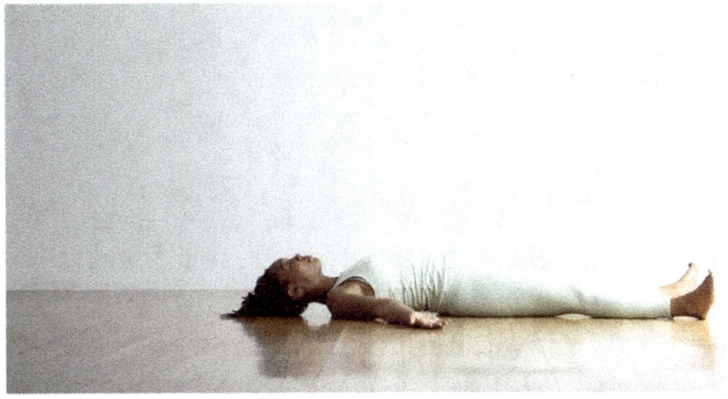

- Tuck your shoulder blades onto your back for support. This is a similar movement to tucking the shoulders under in Bridge Pose, but less intense.
- Once you have set up your limbs, release any effort from holding them in position. Relax your whole body, including your face. Let your body feel heavy.
- Let your breathing occur naturally. If your mind wanders, you can bring your attention to your breath but try to just notice it, not deepen it.
- Stay for a minimum of five minutes. Ten minutes is better. If you are practicing at home, set an alarm so that you are not compelled to keep checking the time.
- To come out, first begin to the deepen your breath. Then begin to wiggle your fingers and toes, slowly reawakening your body.
- Stretch your arms overhead for a full body stretch from hands to feet.
- Bring your knees into your chest and roll over to one side, keeping your eyes closed.
- Use your bottom arm as a pillow while you rest in a fetal position7 for a few breaths.
- Using your hands for support, bring yourself back up into a sitting position.

Things to Keep in Mind

- **Difficulty Doing Nothing**

Teachers often say that Savasana is the most difficult yoga pose, which is really a way of saying that it's really hard for some people to do nothing for 10 minutes.

If you find it challenging, try scanning your body from toe to head, saying the name of each body part and then releasing it. Your body needs this time to absorb the new information it has received through the physical practice.

- **Active Mind**

Often, the mind wants to stay active even when the body is relaxed. Your mind might have been calm during your pose sequence, but now you need to develop that same calmness when at rest. If your mind won't stop chattering, try the basic meditation techniques of noticing your thoughts, labeling them as thinking, and then letting them go.8 Just like other types of yoga, this takes practice. Eventually, you will notice that when your body goes into Savasana, your mind also assumes a relaxed state.

RECLINING BOUND ANGLE WITH BOLSTER

Benefits & Purposes

There are many benefits of supta baddha konasana, including:

- Relieves stress and tension: This pose is very calming and relaxing. It can help to relieve stress and tension from the mind and body.
- Stretches the inner thighs and groin: This pose helps to stretch the inner thighs and groin muscles.
- Opens the hips: This pose helps to open up the hips and release any tightness in the hip area.
- Improves digestion: This pose massages the digestive organs and can help to improve digestion.
- Relieves back pain: This pose can help to relieve back pain by stretching the back muscles.

Directions

- For this pose, you'll need a bolster, a rolled-up blanket, and two yoga blocks to support you.
- To begin, sit up tall on your yoga mat with your legs straight out in front of you.
- Bend your knees and bring the soles of your feet together. Allow your knees to fall out to the sides. If they don't touch the floor, place yoga blocks under your knees to support them.

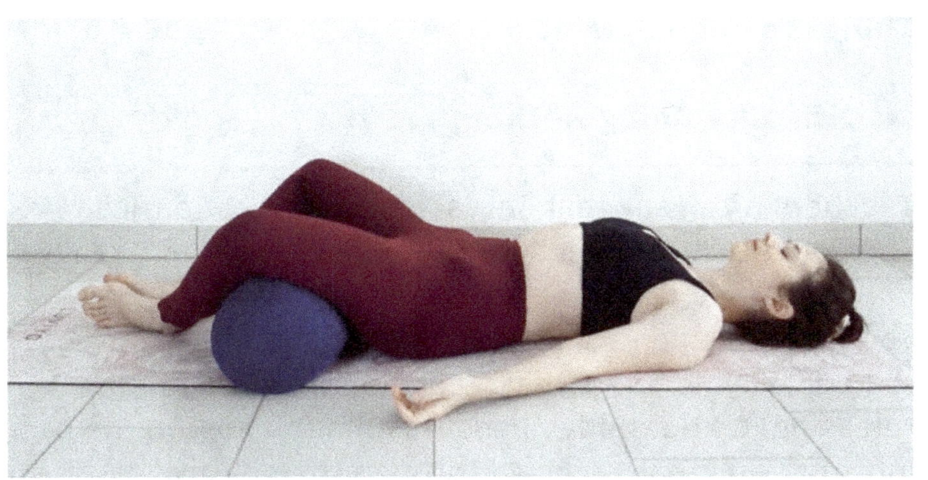

- Place a bolster behind you. The bolster will support the length of your spine, so have one end of it close to your tailbone. The other end of it points behind you. Gently lay back on the bolster.
- You can place a rolled-up blanket or towel beneath your neck to support your head.
- Place your hands at your side or wherever they feel comfortable.
- Stay in this position for 5-10 minutes, breathing deeply and relaxing into the pose.

In conclusion, the supported supta baddha konasana is a great yoga pose for beginners. It is a relaxing and restorative pose that can help relieve stress and tension. This pose can also help to stretch the inner thighs and groin muscles, open up the hips, and improve digestion.

- Use your bottom arm as a pillow while you rest in a fetal position7 for a few breaths.
- Using your hands for support, bring yourself back up into a sitting position.

Things to Keep in Mind

- **Difficulty Doing Nothing**

Teachers often say that Savasana is the most difficult yoga pose, which is really a way of saying that it's really hard for some people to do nothing for 10 minutes. If you find it challenging, try scanning your body from toe to head, saying the name of each body part and then releasing it. Your body needs this time to absorb the new information it has received through the physical practice.

- **Active Mind**

Often, the mind wants to stay active even when the body is relaxed. Your mind might have been calm during your pose sequence, but now you need to develop that same calmness when at rest. If your mind won't stop chattering, try the basic meditation techniques of noticing your thoughts, labeling them as thinking, and then letting them go.8 Just like other types of yoga, this takes practice. Eventually, you will notice that when your body goes into Savasana, your mind also assumes a relaxed state.

LEGS UP THE WALL POSE

Benefits & Purposes

There are many benefits of supta baddha konasana, including:

- Relieves stress and tension: This pose is very calming and relaxing. It can help to relieve stress and tension from the mind and body.
- Stretches the inner thighs and groin: This pose helps to stretch the inner thighs and groin muscles.
- Opens the hips: This pose helps to open up the hips and release any tightness in the hip area.
- Improves digestion: This pose massages the digestive organs and can help to improve digestion.
- Relieves back pain: This pose can help to relieve back pain by stretching the back muscles.

Directions

You may place a cushion, folded blanket, or bolster under your hips. Using a higher support requires more flexibility, as does placing your hips closer to the wall. Adjust accordingly to find your sweet spot.

Bend your knees as much as you like, and if it creates comfort, you can even place a pillow between your knees and the wall.

To draw your attention inward in a practice known as pratyahara, you may wish to cover your eyes using a mask or pillow.

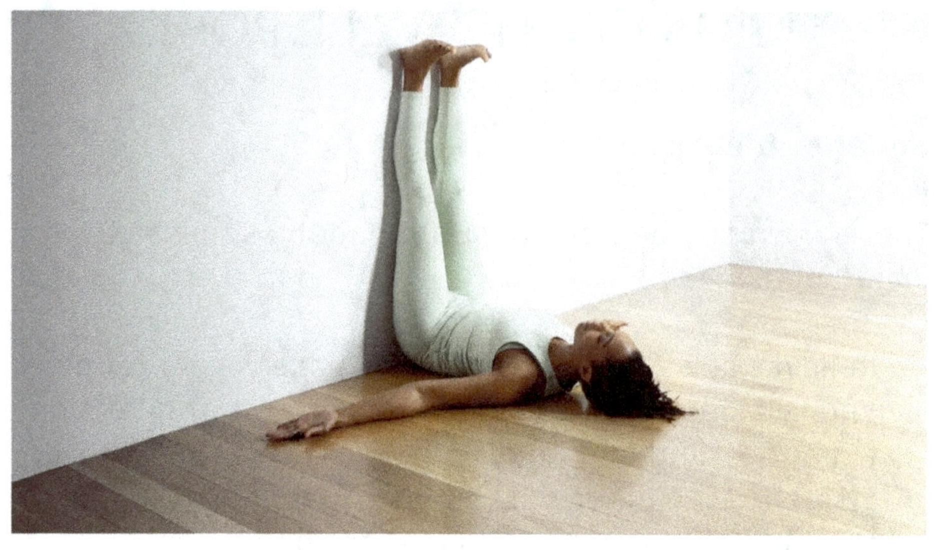

- Sit with your right side against the wall, with bent knees and your feet drawn in toward your hips.
- Swing your legs up against the wall as you turn to lie flat on your back.
- Place your hips against the wall or slightly away.
- Place your arms in any comfortable position.
- Stay in this position for up to 20 minutes.
- To release the pose, gently push yourself away from the wall.
- Relax on your back for a few moments.
- Draw your knees into your chest and roll onto your right side.
- Rest for a few moments before slowly moving into an upright position.

Things to Keep in Mind

It's a gentle posture that can be practiced by just about anyone, anytime, anywhere—as long as you have something to place your legs up onto!

These tips will help protect yourselves from injury and help them have the best experience of the pose:

Place blankets under your head and hips to receive the full benefit of this pose. Fold one blanket into a large square, and then fold it again into thirds, placing it under your hips about 12 inches away from the wall. Fold a second blanket to be used for cushioning your head in half, and place it about 3 feet away from the wall.

As an inversion pose, many benefits come from inverting your notion of "work." The benefits derive not just from inverting an action but also from inverting the whole notion of action. When you relax with your legs up the wall, you are practicing the polar opposite of activity, which is receptivity.

RAG DOLL POSE

Benefits & Purposes

- Stretches the ankles, calves, hamstrings and lower back.
- Releases tension in the neck and shoulders.
- Can help to alleviate lower back and neck pain.
- Relieves stress.

Directions

- Set-Up: Stand with your feet hip width apart, toes pointing forward.
- Action: Inhale, bring your hands to your hips. Exhale, micro-bend your knees and hinge forward from the hips with a flat back. Cross your arms and hold onto opposite elbows.
- Refinements: Check that your knees point straight ahead and that your thighs are parallel. Sway gently from side to side. If you have tight hamstrings, keep your knees bent to avoid straining your lower back. If that still feels like a lot of pressure at your lower back, rest your hands on a block to support the weight of your upper body.
- Standing Forward Bend: If you are safe to straighten your legs, contract your quadriceps to allow your hamstrings to relax. You can take hold of the backs of your calves, bring your hands to the floor or wrap your fingers and thumbs around your big toes.
- Duration: Hold the pose for 3-5 deep breaths, in and out through the nose.

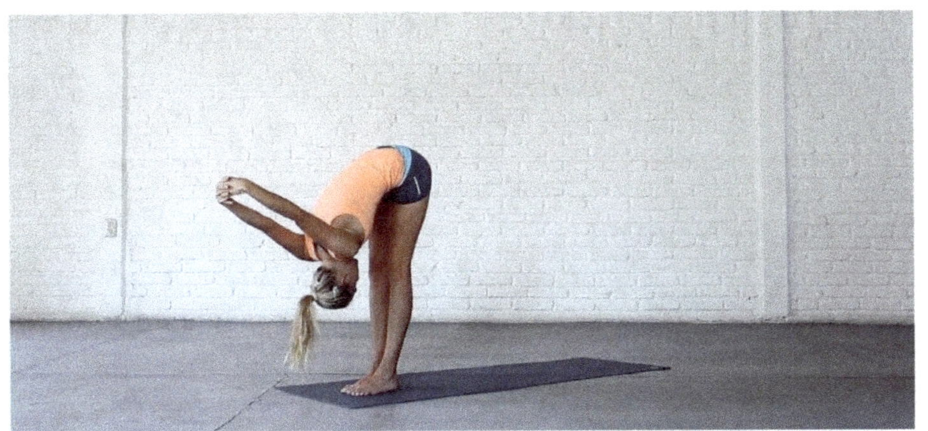

- To Release: To come out of the pose, bring your hands to your hips, keep the micro-bend in your knees and come up to standing with a flat back— engaging your core to support your lower back.

Things to Keep in Mind

Although this pose stretches the entire back body, the focus is on the back and not the hamstrings. Therefore, you can bend your knees generously. This will allow your chest to connect to the thighs, and consequently, the back will relax more. You can use props to deepen the stretch – e.g. lean the back on a wall or step your toes on a folded blanket.

In yin yoga, this pose is held for 3 minutes or more, but that can be too difficult. You can perform it in several shorter, one or two-minute sessions, and enter Garland Pose (Yogi Squat) between the reps. Swaying side to side and front to back can help you release tension and stabilize yourself in the pose – check how this movement changes the sensation in the feet. Find a place where your weight is centered between the balls of the feet and the heels.

ONE-LEGGED SEATED FORWARD BEND

Benefits & Purposes

Seated One-Legged Forward Fold gives a nice stretch in the back legs, from the glutes, to the hamstrings then to the calves and is also a good stretch for the side body — from the armpits to the ribcage then to the hip. It massages the internal organs with each concentrated breath, which then stimulates good digestion.

As with any hamstring stretch, practicing this asana will release low back pain. This pose is also very calming for the mind, alleviating any stress or anxiety from the everyday demands of life.

Directions

- Sit on the floor with your legs stretched out straight in front of you, keeping your spine erect.
- Bend your left knee and place your left foot against your right thigh, keeping your left knee on the floor.
- Breathing in, raise both arms above your head and stretch up. Twist slightly to the right from your waist.
- Breathing out, bend forward from your hip joints, keeping the spine straight and directing your chin to your toes.
- If you can, hold onto your big toes and, pointing your elbows to the ground, move forward as you pull on your toes.

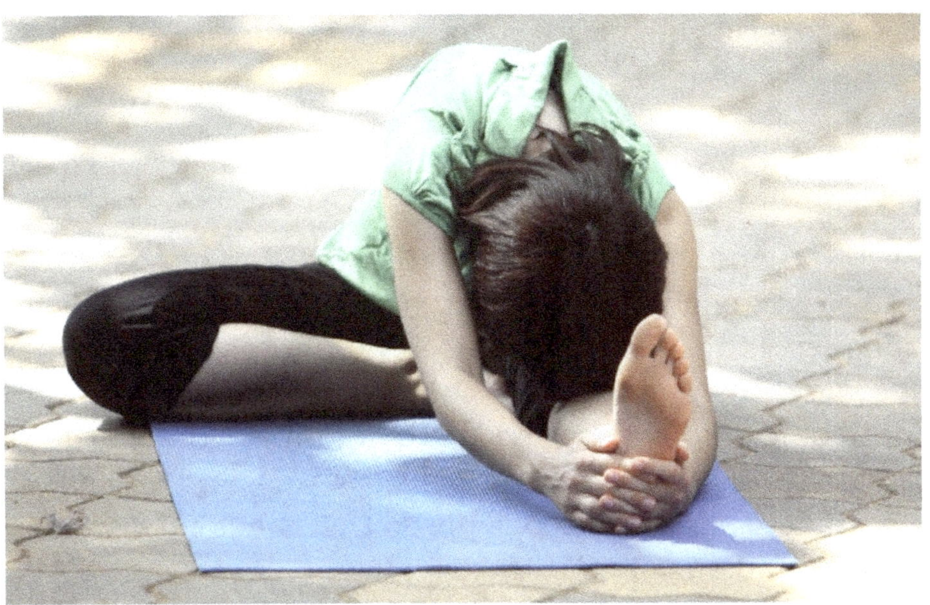

- Hold. Keep breathing.
- Breathing in, come up and breathing out, bring your arms down to your sides.
- Repeat on the other side.

Things to Keep in Mind

While a regular yoga practice can result in improved health, know that it is not a substitute for medical treatment. It is important to learn and practice yoga under the supervision of a trained teacher.

REVOLVED ABDOMEN POSE

Benefits & Purposes

Revolved Abdomen Pose strengthens the spine, back, and all of the abdominal muscles, particularly the obliques. It increases flexibility and reduces stiffness in the spine, lower back, hips, chest, and shoulders. Stretching and twisting the spine not only hydrates the spinal discs, but it also lengthens, relaxes, and realigns the spine. This pose is considered therapeutic for stress, fatigue, and anxiety.

Twisting the spine has many benefits. When the torso is revolved, the organs of digestion and elimination (including the liver, kidneys, and spleen) are compressed. This compression helps these organs release toxins and metabolic waste. When the twist is released, these organs receive a fresh flow of oxygenated blood, which helps them to continue flushing out the toxins. Twists improve the overall health and function of your digestive system.

Directions

- To begin, lie on your back with your knees bent and your feet flat on the floor. You can rest your head on a pillow or blanket.
- Extend your arms out along the floor at shoulder-height with your palms facing down. Straighten your legs, reaching your heels up toward the ceiling.

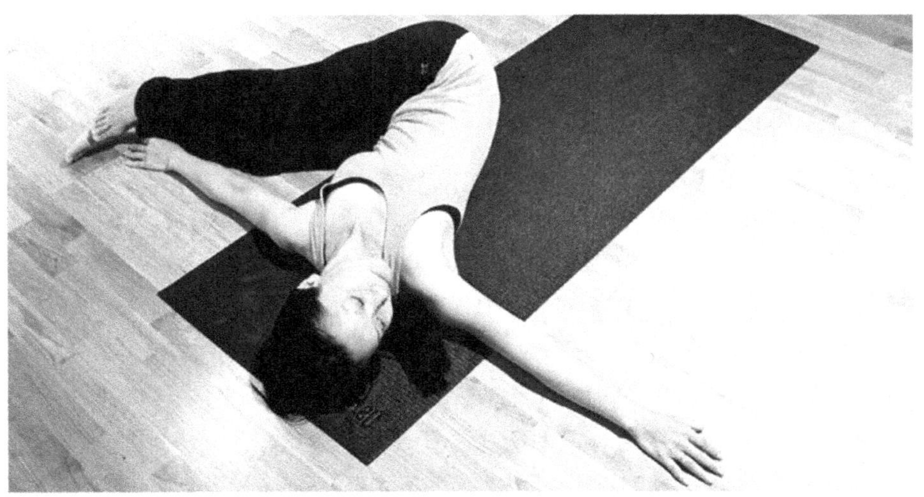

- Align your heels directly over your hips. Keep your knees soft and slightly bent.
- Draw your low back down, so it is flat on the floor. On an exhalation, lower your legs to the left, twisting your spine and allowing your right hip to lift all the way off the floor. Allow the force of gravity to drop your legs all the way down. Allow your left foot to rest on the floor.
- Flex your feet and stack the outer edge of your right ankle on top of your left.
- Work toward bringing your torso and legs into a 90-degree angle, or slightly less. If your legs are angled up toward your left shoulder, you can clasp your left foot's toes with your right hand's fingers.
- Turn your head to the right. Soften your gaze toward your right hand's fingertips. Keep your shoulder blades pressing down toward the floor and away from your ears.
- Hold the pose for 10-25 breaths.

- On an inhalation, slowly come back to center, raising your feet straight up to the ceiling. Bend your knees and hug them to your chest in Knees-to-Chest Pose (Apanasana).
- On an exhalation, reach your heels up to the ceiling again. Repeat steps 3-7 on the opposite side.
- When you're finished with the pose, hug your knees to your chest for a few breaths in Knees-to-Chest Pose (Apanasana). Then slowly exhale as you extend both legs along the floor.

Things to Keep in Mind

Practicing Revolved Abdomen Pose can be calming and soothing, particularly at the end of the day. Keep the following information in mind when practicing this pose:
- For those with back injuries, be sure to consult with a knowledgeable and experienced instructor before attempting this pose.
- Bring your legs or knees over only as much as comfort will allow. If needed, rest your legs on a bolster or pillow to decrease the range of motion.
- Focus on keeping your shoulders on the floor. Relax your shoulders away from your ears.
- Keep your breath smooth and deep. Do not hold your breath.
- Relax your abdominal muscles and let your belly feel hollow.
- Never force your knees to the floor. Be gentle with yourself!
- Be aware of how your back feels during the pose. If you feel any sharp, pinching, or jarring pain, stop the pose and come out of it slowly, but immediately. Never force the twist if you are in pain.

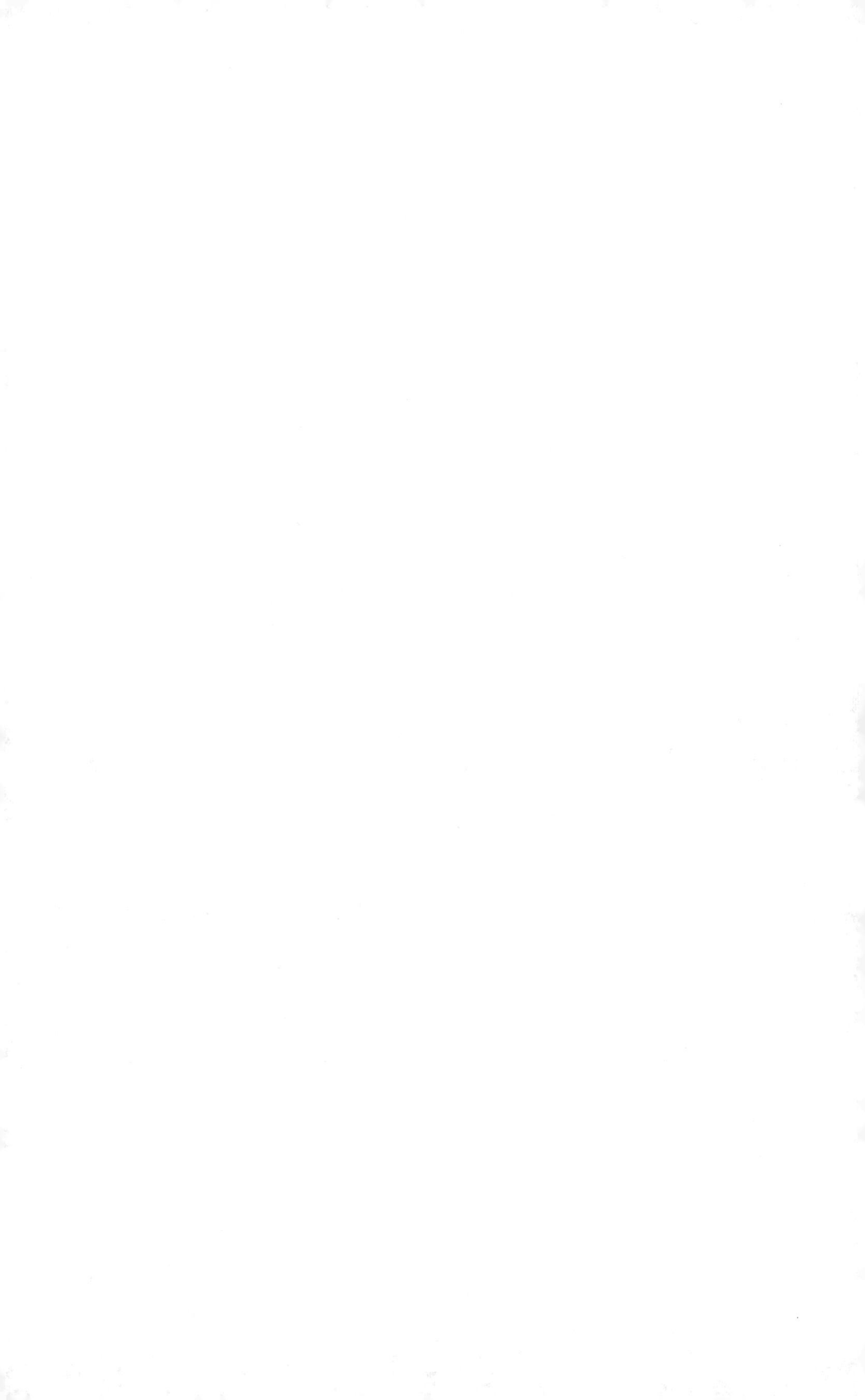

9 7 9 8 3 3 7 5 3 2 2 3 3